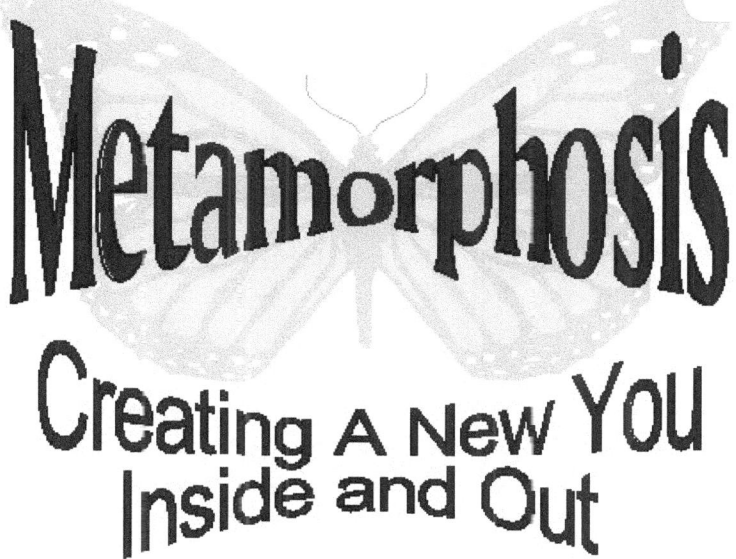

Metamorphosis
Creating A New You Inside and Out

30-Days to No More IDA
(Iron Deficiency Anemia)

By

Allen Lawrence, M.D., M.A., Ph.D.

and

Lisa Robyn Lawrence, M.S., Ph.D.

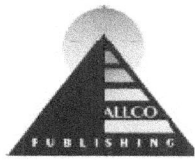

Tarzana, California

Medical Disclaimer

Nothing said within this book is meant to have you make any self diagnosis, alter existing medical treatment nor avoid seeing your doctor for a competent medical evaluation, diagnosis and appropriate treatment.

The sole purpose of this book is to educate the reader and make medical terms available and familiar to those individuals who are interested. If you believe that there is something wrong with you or that you have an unexplained problem involving your health or physical, mental or emotional well-being, then we encourage you to call and make an appointment with your doctor. You should discuss your health concerns with a competent licensed physician who can make an appropriate diagnosis and provide competent treatment for any medical condition that may exist.

The goal of this book is four fold: 1) To educate people in how to recognize iron deficiency anemia and its early symptoms, so that they can seek appropriate medical care as early as is possible. 2) To assist individuals, after the diagnosis of iron deficiency anemia has been made, in choosing healthy iron rich foods which can compliment a physician prescribed treatment program. 3) To assist men, women and children, in selecting foods that will help them in preventing the occurrence of iron deficiency and anemia hence requiring medical treatment. 4) As part of a dietary regime to either prevent or treat iron deficiency anemia during and after pregnancy.

Lastly, the treatment of iron deficiency anemia, depending on its severity may take longer than 30days, however, it should not take longer than 30 days to get started on this program and this program along with medical treatment in an individual with severe iron deficiency anemia should greatly help to improve iron blood levels and assist in treating and reversing the iron deficiency and the associated anemia.

Self diagnosis and treatment can be dangerous. Consult a qualified medical doctor if you are having any problems you are concerned about.

Allen Lawrence, M.D.

Dedication

We dedicate this book to the thousands of people we have directly worked with and treated in our medical practice and for the many thousands of people who have used our website looking for more information, for answers, definitions and help in understanding medical problems they were going through or suffering from.

We hope that this work will help thousands more to understand what is happening to them and why it is happening. We hope to enable people to become better informed and more able to communicate with and understand their doctor's instructions so that their medical conditions are treated most effectively and appropriately.

Introduction

While iron deficiency anemia is rarely fatal it can under certain circumstances be quite disabling and uncomfortable. Year after year one of the more popular web pages on our website *Wellness on the Web* at http://www.well-net.com has consistently been our pages on Foods High in Iron. We also get many questions regarding how to eat a high iron diet. For many years we have answered each question individually, yet clearly all of the questions appear to have a common theme, men and women looking for information for themselves, about their children or even on occasion regarding a partner who suffers from iron deficiency anemia.

While we are always available to answer questions more often then not simply e-mail back and forth is not the absolute best media to present all of the information that is often required. To resolve this we have decided to combine all of the questions we have been asked, along with basic information most people with iron deficiency anemia wish to have answered. We have added tables and lists of foods that contain iron or promote easy resolution of iron deficiency anemia into a short yet information packed book.

We now offer this book to those individuals who wish to have answers to those questions which are most important to them about the causes, reasons for, medical treatment and supportive measures they can take to aid in preventing and treating iron deficiency anemia. We now offer this book to all readers who have questions and need solutions regarding iron deficiency anemia.

Allen Lawrence, M.D., Ph.D.
Lisa Robyn Lawrence, M.S., Ph.D.

Table Of Contents

Warnings

The treatment of any iron preparation should always be under the care, advice and supervision of a legally licenced physician. Since iron products interfere with absorption of oral tetracycline antibiotics, these products should not be taken within 2 hours of each other. As with any drug, if you are pregnant or nursing a baby, seek the advice of a health professional before using this product. Accidental overdose of iron-containing products is a leading cause of fatal poisoning in children under 6 years of age, there fore it is important to KEEP THESE PRODUCTS OUT OF REACH OF CHILDREN. In case of accidental overdose, call a doctor or poison control center immediately.

(This Page Is Purposefully Left Blank For You To Use To Take Notes)

Chapter 1

Do You Need More Iron In Your Diet?

What Is Iron?

Iron is one of the many essential minerals. It is a metal, which is necessary for human life and well-being. Iron is officially designated as *Fe* on the Periodic Table of Elements, but in fact there are two types of iron, Ferrous iron (Fe^{++} or heme iron) and Ferric iron (Fe^{+++} which is also known as non-heme iron). Without iron we could not exist as we do, nor could we live for very long. Iron's most important role is found within our red blood cells where iron joins with a protein molecule to form a chemical compound called *hemoglobin*. Hemoglobin in turn binds with oxygen and carries oxygen throughout our body releasing oxygen where and when it is needed to ensure our ability to function optimally.

Within our body iron is considered to be a trace mineral. This means there is only a very small amount of it at any one time. When an individual becomes depleted of sufficient iron to make adequate hemoglobin, that individual is said to have or even suffer from *iron deficiency anemia* or IDA.

What Is IDA?

Iron deficiency is the most common known form of nutritional deficiency. It is also the most common cause of anemia worldwide. Nine percent of infants and toddlers and about 10% of adolescent girls and women of child-bearing age are iron deficient. IDA is generally uncommon in adult males.

IDA occurs when we have a shortage of the heme form of iron in our body, and we are therefore unable to either make a sufficient amount or quality of hemoglobin to carry adequate amounts of oxygen for our bodily needs. Ultimately this creates either a decreased amount or decreased quality of hemoglobin and this translates into either 1) a decreased number of red blood cells being manufactured, or 2) a decrease in the amount of hemoglobin within each red blood cell. Iron is also important because it plays an essential role in energy production for the body. It is essential in the formation and use of several enzymes and proteins. Iron also plays an important role in protection against the effects of stress, the proper functioning of the immune system and in our overall well-being.

No matter the cause (and there a number of causes), IDA can create health problems which can negatively affect us and reduce the quality of our life. At its very extreme it can on occasion, be fatal. We shall, in the remainder of this book, discuss the milder and obviously non-fatal consequences of IDA.

Anemia occurs most commonly in young children (especially, those under two years of age), teenage girls, women of childbearing age, pregnant and breast feeding women and the elderly. In children, iron deficiency and IDA can cause developmental delays and long-term behavioral problems. In pregnant women, it increases the risk of a preterm onset of labor and delivering a below normal birth weight baby. While in the general population, periodic screening has helped reduce the total numbers of individuals suffering from chronic anemia, in women of childbearing age, iron deficiency has remained a significant problem.

How Does IDA Occur?

There are many reasons why someone can become anemic due to iron deficiency. The most common reasons are:

- Eating a diet which is deficient in iron:

  ‣ Inadequate diet, a diet which is deficient in available iron
  ‣ Strict vegetarian diets (primarily non-heme iron diets)
  ‣ Lower income people who cannot afford or obtain an adequate diet
  ‣ Pica, which is clay, ice or paper chewing (Chapter 4, Special Situations, Pica)
  ‣ Chronic dieting, especially with calorie restricted diets, but also bulimia and purging

- Increased requirements for iron beyond that available normally in a diet which contains adequate amounts of iron:

  ‣ Blood loss (excessive menstruation, hemorrhoids, peptic ulcer, cancer of the bowel, etc.)
  ‣ Inadequate digestion, poor hydrochloric acid production. This is more common in middle-aged women and elderly, men and women alike.
  ‣ Prolonged use of antacids (because of indigestion or peptic ulcer disease), sufficient

hydrochloric acid must be present in the stomach in order for iron to be absorbed.
- A diet which is either too high in or deficient of vitamins, minerals or other compounds or foods which either compete with, normally enhance or reduce the absorption of iron into the body (see phytates and oxylates Chapter 3).

  - A diet deficient in vitamin C
  - Excessive calcium (such as dairy products or supplements) may decrease iron absorption, leading to IDA (the addition of even a modest amount of milk or cheese to a meal of pizza or hamburger has been shown to reduce iron absorption by 50-60%).
  - High intake of phosphorus-containing foods (such as in carbonated soft drinks and extremely high protein diets) can interfere with iron absorption.
  - Tannic acid is found in commercial black and pekoe teas, coffee, cola drinks, chocolate, and red wines. Excessive intake of coffee (even decaffeinated coffee, can reduce iron uptake as much as 39%), tea (can reduce iron uptake as much as 87%), or red wine (excessive polyphenols).
  - High levels of phytic acid, a compound found in rye bread, beans (legumes) and other foods made from whole grains as well as in nonherbal teas.
  - Deficient intake of copper, manganese, cobalt, molybdenum, vitamins A, vitamin D and the B vitamins (especially riboflavin, vitamin B2). All of these vitamins and minerals are essential for complete iron absorption and adequate iron uptake. When any or all of these vitamins and minerals are insufficient or deficient in the diet, iron up-take and absorption can be significantly reduced.
  - Excessive amounts of zinc and vitamin E, like calcium mentioned above, can interfere with iron absorption.
  - Another inhibitor of iron absorption includes the common preservative EDTA

- Medications which can interfere with iron absorption NSAID's (non-steroidal anti-inflammatory medications), aspirin and tetracycline, which is often used to treat acne or infection, can interfere with iron absorption.
- Growth spurts create a greater need for iron.
- Athletes or those who exercise regularly and strenuously, especially long distance runners.
- Teenagers, especially those with poor diet and newly menstruating young women.
- The elderly (especially those who eat a poor or inadequate diet).
- A decreased ability to absorb iron from the digestive system (see above).
- Pregnancy, loss of iron to the baby and increase need for iron as blood volume expands.
- Breast feeding, increased loss of iron into breast milk.
- Blood loss from the gastrointestinal tract, bleeding ulcers, GI tumors, hookworms.
- Blood loss from heavy menstrual periods.
- Decreased iron absorption after stomach or small bowel surgery.
- Excessive blood donation or blood testing.

> ► Chronic infection, any type
> ► Chronic gum disease

- Medical problems such as heart valve disease, other types of anemia, loss of iron into the tissues of the body, loss of hemoglobin in the urine, cancer, rheumatoid arthritis, candidiasis or chronic herpes infections

- Infants and babies may become iron deficient because:
  - ► Their diet is deficient in adequate iron caused by unsupplemented cow's milk only diets
  - ► Breast feeding, mother is deficient in sufficient iron to enrich her breast milk
  - ► Toddlers and children can become iron deficient if their daily diet is deficient or improperly balanced, when there is inadequate iron to meet their growth needs and for making adequate red blood cells.

One of the more important reasons for IDA is blood loss, especially from the gastrointestinal tract. Chronic usage of aspirin can cause chronic blood loss and therefore iron loss, even without an ulcer or visible bleeding from the gastrointestinal tract. Unexplained iron deficiency should suggest an immediate search for any potential source of gastrointestinal bleeding once all other sources of blood loss have been eliminated (heavy menstrual periods, other reasons for uterine bleeding, and repeated blood donations).

Another group of people who are frequently at risk for IDA are strict "Vegan" vegetarians (those who do not consume any animal products) and those vegetarians who eat an inadequate unbalanced diet. As with non-vegetarians pregnant or lactating women or women with heavy menstrual losses, those with chronic blood losses caused by conditions such as gastric ulcers or intestinal tumors are at even greater risk.

Many times the first sign of a malignant intestinal tumor is IDA.

Another reason for IDA is decreased iron absorption because of vitamin-mineral imbalance or past stomach surgery.

Chronic loss of blood or hemoglobin in the urine(hemoglobinuria) can also produce a state of iron deficiency, since more than 1 mg each day of iron can be lost through this route. The most common cause is traumatic hemolysis due to an abnormally functioning cardiac valve, usually mechanical and prosthetic. Other causes of intravascular hemolysis (e.g., paroxysmal nocturnal hemoglobinuria) should also be considered if hemoglobinuria is documented.

A rare cause of iron deficiency can be idiopathic pulmonary hemosiderosis where iron is selectively stored in certain cells within the lungs.

How Much Iron Do We Need

The average person has a total of somewhere between 2 grams and 4 grams of iron in his or her body. The average woman is likely to have about 2.5 grams of iron in total, while the average man would contain about 3.8 grams total of iron within his body. Between 70% and 95% of this iron is found in the hemoglobin[1] which makes up the red blood cells circulating throughout our body. Apart from the iron circulating in the red blood cells, there are also several major iron storage pools. These storage pools consists of supplies of iron which are deposited and held in reserve for the future. The pools lie within specific bodily tissues. Such as within the large muscles of the body, certain cells in the lungs, the liver, and in the marrow of the long bone. In these areas iron is either stored in the form of a chemical called *ferritin*[2], or as *hemosiderin*[3], or are located in special cells of the immune system called *macrophages*[4]. Iron is moved from one part of the body to another within blood by the protein transferrin. The range for storage of iron can be quite broad and usually varies greatly from person to person. Studies have shown however, that approximately 25% of all women in the US actually have little or no identifiable iron reserves in their body. That is, they have no stored iron, only the iron actively being used for hemoglobin or other purposes in within their body.

As you can see, we humans do not contain very large amounts of iron, yet iron is still essential to our ability to live and stay healthy. Even small amounts of deficiency can lead to large problems.

How Much Iron Do We Need?

Our body has many ways of conserving iron. When red blood cells are destroyed, the iron inside them is reused in the production of new red blood cells. However, there is a daily iron loss approximately 1 mg a day, which normally must be replenished by our daily diet.

The first and most important answer to this question is we need enough iron to make sufficient hemoglobin. Next we need enough iron to take care of all of the other roles iron plays in our body. Thirdly we need enough iron to meet our daily loss of iron because of natural causes (this will be discussed in greater detail in a later section). All of that said, then how much iron do we need on a daily basis to make sure all of these needs are taken care of?

The US Department of Agriculture suggests a Recommended Dietary Allowance (RDA) for adults of 10 to 18 mg of iron per day in our diet. See Table 1, below for specific details by age.

Who Is Most Likely to Develop IDA ? - The Incidence of IDA.

● The occurrence of iron deficiency is greatest among toddlers aged 1-2 years (about 7% of all toddlers) and adolescents and adults, mostly women, aged 12-49 years (9%-16%).

As you can see from the reasons people become iron deficient, and from the statistics above, women and children are most likely to develop IDA. Women become deficient because of their dietary deficiencies in iron and because of menstruation. Children also develop IDA primarily because of inadequate iron in their diet. In men, the most common reason for anemia is chronic loss of blood from the gastrointestinal tract. The exact reason why iron is often deficient in the diet will become more clear as you read on. We will discuss the role of diet in creating and healing IDA in a later section.

RDA's For Iron

Females ages 11-50	15 mg
Females - pregnant*	30 mg
Females - lactation*	15 mg
Females ages 50+	10 mg
Males ages 11-18	12 mg
Males, adult	10 mg
Infants 0-6 months	10 mg
Children 6 mo-10 yrs	6 mg

*requires supplementation

Table 1

Where Do We Get Our Iron From?

You have probably already recognized that iron primarily enters into our body from the foods we eat. The average American diet will provide about 10 mg to 15 mg of iron each day when eaten according to the Food Pyramid Guide (See Figure 2). Only about 10% of this iron can be absorbed into our body. When we eat iron rich foods more iron is absorbed through our stomach and upper intestinal tract. When the dietary iron is present as the heme (or ferrous) form of iron the most that can be effectively absorbed is only about 10%. Under good circumstances your body may even be able to absorb up to a maximum of 20% of the iron available to the digestive system. When the diet is made up primarily of non-heme (defined below) sources of iron, then significantly less iron will likely be absorbed, somewhere between only 1% and 5% at most. The *bioavailability* (our ability to absorb iron) of this non-heme iron can be strongly affected by the other foods ingested within the same meal. Competing nutrients such as phosphates, polyphenols (in certain vegetables), tannins (in tea), phytates (in bran), oxylates, and calcium (in dairy products) and other food constituents in the diet can limit non-heme iron absorption. On the other hand, absorption of non-heme iron can be increased by having an adequate amount of vitamin C (fruits and some vegetables) in our diet.

Our ability to absorb iron from our diet will also depend on four conditions:

1. The amount of iron already in our body
2. The rate that red blood cells are produced by our body
3. The amount and kinds of iron in our diet, and
4. the presence of absorption enhancers or inhibitors within our diet.

Our gastrointestinal tract increases its ability to absorb iron when our body's iron stores are low. It will also decrease our ability to absorb iron when these stores are abundant. An increased rate of red blood cell production can also stimulate iron uptake from what we eat. Absorption of iron generally increases during pregnancy, however this increase is not always very well defined and can be irregular. After delivering a baby iron stores tend to increase and iron absorption tends to decrease.

Iron Turnover and Loss

Generally, most people eat a relatively healthy iron rich diet. Their iron metabolism is easily balanced between their absorption of 1 mg of iron each day and their loss of 1 mg of iron each day. When illness, nutritional deficiencies, heavy menstrual periods, gastrointestinal bleeding and pregnancy occur this balance can be rapidly upset. When this happens the daily intake of iron must be increased up to 2 mg a day. Sometimes an increase as high as 5 mg of iron daily may be necessary in those individuals where the out-go of iron is greater than their usual intake of iron. When this happens maintaining the usual dietary intake of iron may not meet their increased need for iron. Since most people are not extremely sophisticated regarding which foods contain iron, or which are iron rich and which foods and chemicals will likely interfere with iron absorption, medicinal iron is often resorted to as the best way to treat this loss and increased need. This is especially true during pregnancy and breast feeding. When women experience repeat pregnancies without replenishing their lost iron stores (especially when they are also breast feeding), this may further worsen iron deficiency. These women often require both an increase in dietary iron intake along with iron supplementation.

In women menstruation plays a major role in iron metabolism. The average monthly blood loss from menstruation is approximately about 0.7 mg of iron each day of bleeding. However, menstrual blood loss can be as much as five times this average in some women. In any individual woman, during any cycle, or for a day or two of heavy bleeding, a greater than normal loss of blood and iron can occur. In order to maintain adequate iron stores, women with heavy menstrual blood losses must ingest and absorb 3 mg to 4 mg of iron each and every day of their adult life. This amount often strains the upper limit of what may be easily absorbed, and women with heavier than average menstrual bleeding are frequently iron-deficient.

The formation of red blood cells and their destruction is responsible for most of the turnover of iron in our body. The red blood cells which carry iron-rich hemoglobin can live for only 120 days or about four months. Unless there is a continual supply of iron, vitamin B12, vitamin C and folacin from either food or supplements, first depletion of iron stores will occur. If this level of iron deficiency is not corrected the result will be poorly formed red blood cells that are ineffective carrying adequate amounts of oxygen to the body. This then will end up leading to some or all of the various symptoms of IDA.

In adult men, more than 95% of the iron required in the production of red blood cells is recycled iron obtained from the breakdown of older red blood cells. Only 5% of iron in this case will end up coming from the diet. On the other hand, in infants it is estimated that nearly 70% of red blood cell iron comes from the breakdown of older red blood cells and 30% comes from the infant's diet.

Dietary Intake of Iron

The best source of prevention of IDA is a good healthy balanced diet. If you are at risk for IDA or already have mild to moderate IDA, iron-rich foods are your best form of treatment. Foods with the highest sources of available iron (heme iron) are primarily animal products such as meat, milk, and eggs. Vegetables such as spinach and broccoli have a large amount of (non-heme) iron, but the intestine is often unable to easily absorb iron from these sources.

> **Heme iron**, that is iron found only in meat, poultry, and fish, is between two to three times more absorbable than **non-heme iron**, which is found in plant-based foods and iron-fortified foods.

What Are the Most Common Signs and Symptoms of IDA?

As a rule, the primary symptoms of IDA are those which are directly related to the anemia itself. Generally, low or even depleted iron stores do nct express any symptoms or signs. Only when there is greater than the mildest anemia, will symptoms or signs occur. The most common symptoms of IDA are:

Signs and symptoms of mild IDA:

- No symptoms at all or possibly only,
- Feeling tired, fatigued or easy fatigability
- Sensitivity to cold
- Increased frequency of colds, flu or other viral infections

Signs and symptoms of moderate to mildly severe IDA:

- Rapid pulse (tachycardia)
- Irregular heart beat (palpitations)
- Shortness of breath on exertion (tachypnea)
- Brittle hair
- Difficulty with digestion
- Nervousness
- Headaches
- Impaired concentration
- Impaired physical capacity and ability to work
- Decrease in immune functions, increasing the chance of various illnesses and of infection.
- Weight gain and even obesity
- Restless legs syndrome (uncomfortable feeling in legs, sensations of pulling, tingling or crawling), accompanied by a need to move the legs

Signs and symptoms of moderately severe to severe IDA:

- Skin or changes in mucous membranes (mouth, nose vagina)
- A smoothing of the tongue
- Nails become brittle
- Sores, redness, fissures (cracks or splits in the skin) at the sides or corners of the mouth (cheilosis)
- Difficulty swallowing (dysphagia) is a rare finding of severe IDA.
- Behavioral and cognitive problems

- In extreme cases, shortness of breath

In adults IDA can impair an individual's capacity to work and function at work as well as in their day-to-day life. Fortunately these impairments appear to be at least partially reversible once iron treatment has replenished the iron deficiency. It is not yet known whether IDA can affect an individual's capacity to perform less physically demanding labor which is dependent on sustained clarity of mind or coordinated motor functions.

Iron Toxicity- Too Much Iron

- Infections
- Hemochromatosis (se below), an iron metabolism disorder resulting in failure of multiple organ systems
- Liver damage
- Possible increased risk of cancer and heart disease risk
- Death

Iron toxicity is rare from dietary sources, however, toxicity can easily occur from use of iron medications or supplements. This is especially true if they are misused and not used according to the instructions on the product label. We will continually stress that children can very easily be poisoned by iron. When iron supplements or medications are in the home they should be put in places that are higher enough and out of the way where children can reach them or they should be locked up.

How Is the Diagnosis of IDA Made?

The simplest way to make a diagnosis of IDA is through physical examination and basic laboratory testing to confirm and determine the severity of the anemia. Often the individual with IDA is pale, their nail beds and oral mucous membranes are pale and not their usual bright pink. Often the medical history is a give away as the anemic individual (especially with moderate to severe anemia) will likely complain of fatigue or inability to perform daily work. They may complain, "I no longer have my old reserve of energy!" "I am tired all of the time!" When the anemia is more severe then the other symptoms of IDA, as they are listed above, may be found. There is frequently a history of some reason for blood loss. One very common example in women is heavier than normal menstrual periods, multiple pregnancies, breast-feeding, recent c-section delivery or other surgery. Any individual with gastrointestinal bleeding, no matter the reason, having black stools or black tar-like stools, should be evaluated for gastrointestinal bleeding.

What Diagnostic Laboratory Testing Might My Doctor Order For Me?

IDA generally develops in stages (see Table 2). In the earliest stages there is a slow depletion of iron stores and reserves from the body tissues. This generally occurs along with a mild state of anemia. At this point there is generally no physical changes involving the size or shape of the red blood cells. Even after iron stores have been significantly depleted the creation of red blood cells will continue even though the iron stores are deficient. Red cell production occurs if there is at least an adequate intake of iron in the diet. However, as iron stores are depleted and if there are inadequate amounts of iron in the diet on a daily basis, the formation of red blood cells will gradually be affected. Once depletion is severe and diet is not improved red cell production will first create small, microcytic cells with little iron in them and eventually stop making red blood cells in adequate amounts.

Once anemia of any type is suspected, after the medical history and physical examination has been performed your doctor will likely order a simple blood test called a CBC or *cellular blood count*. This is the most common method of confirming the diagnosis of anemia (of all types). This test may also indicate that this is IDA. This blood test will initially be evaluated for the amount of hemoglobin in the sample and a hematocrit test is performed. The hematocrit test is also a simple test. A small amount of whole unclotted blood is spun down and the ratio of the newly packed red blood cells to the remaining blood plasma is easily measured. This is read as a percentage of red blood cells versus plasma. A normal hematocrit in an adult female should be greater than 35%. Next a series of evaluations called *indices* are performed. These indices include the *mean corpuscular volume* (MCV)[5], *mean corpuscular hemoglobin* (MCH)[6] and *mean corpuscular hemoglobin concentration* (MCHC)[7]. Finally a drop of blood is examined under a microscope. This is usually referred to as a *blood smear*. A drop or two of blood is smeared out on the face of a glass slide and a technician looks under his microscope at the smears and specifically at the red blood cells to determine their size, shape and other specific characteristics (See Figure 1).

As the anemia progresses the MCV will eventually begin to fall and a blood smear will show small, pale red blood cells called *hypochromic microcytic cells*[8]. These small hypochromic cells are characteristic of IDA. As the anemia worsens the size of the red blood cells will begin to vary greatly (a condition referred to as *anisocytosis*). More cells will become small, however some will remain normal in size, and some may even become slightly larger than normal. Eventually the shape of these iron deficient red cells will begin to vary (a condition called *poikilocytosis*). As the anemia progresses these variations will become more significant and more obvious in the required blood tests.

In severe IDA there is often a quite bizarre appearing blood smear with severely hypochromic cells, abnormal cells called *target cells*, hypochromic pencil-shaped cells, and occasionally small numbers of very young and primitive *nucleated red blood cells*. The number and shape of the blood platelets (involved in the clotting mechanism of the body) are generally normal in mild IDA but will begin to vary and become distorted as the anemia progresses. As IDA advances the platelet count may become increasingly abnormal as well.

Sometimes, especially when the diagnosis is not clear, other much more specific (and costly) tests may need to be performed in order to make or confirm the diagnosis of IDA and rule out all other types of anemias. One of these special tests is the blood chemical test, *serum ferritin*[2]. In very mild anemia serum ferritin may be entirely normal, however as the anemia progresses with time, the total amount of serum ferritin will gradually become lower and lower until it is abnormally low. When serum ferritin reaches a value of less than 30 µg/L it nearly always becomes an excellent indicator that iron stores are significantly depleted and is therefore a very reliable indicator of iron deficiency. Another test that may be used is *serum total iron-binding capacity* (TIBC), TIBC is also known as *transferrin saturation*[9], and in IDA it will eventually fall to less than 15% in severe iron deficiency, this will be discussed briefly below). As the anemia progresses the TIBC will begin to rise slowly at first but steadily in relation to the depletion of iron stores in the body.

Stages of Iron Deficiency Anemia			
Stage	**Change**	**What Happens**	**Diagnostic Test to Evaluate**
Stage I	**Depletion of Iron Reserves and Stores**	Occurs over time, because of an iron deficient diet, excessive bleeding or other causes for depletion of iron stores. There are generally no external manifestations of this depletion.	Serum ferritin Bone marrow iron
Stage II	**Production of Iron Deficient Red Blood Cells**	As iron stores fall, normal red blood cells cannot be made. Cells are deficient in hemoglobin and hence gradually reduced in size. Red blood cells are made with flaws during their manufacturing process not only smaller than normal but in irregular shapes and sizes	Serum ferritin Bone marrow iron Serum iron TIBC

Stage III	Iron Deficiency Anemia	Red blood cells are decreased in number, irregular size and shape, smaller than normal in size and often have hollowed-out centers .	Serum ferritin Bone marrow iron Serum iron TIBC Hemoglobin Hematocrit MCV RDW

Table 2

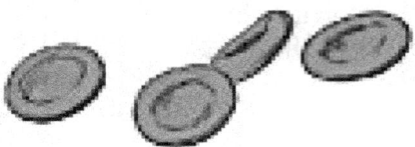

Red Blood Cells in Anemia

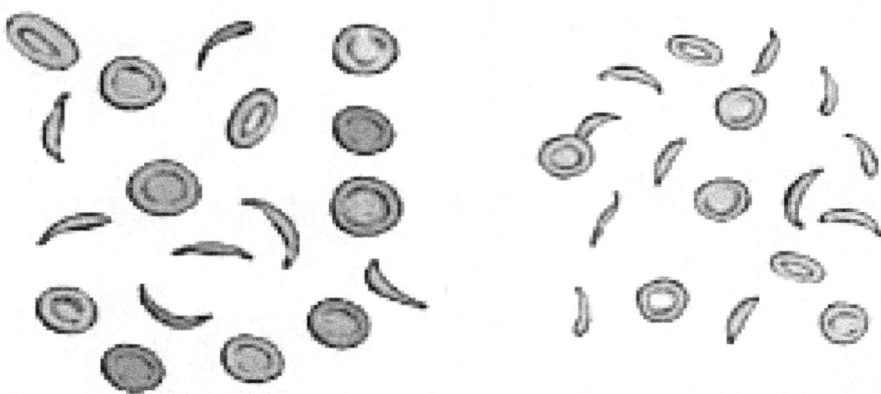

Healthy "Normal" Red Blood Cells

Mild to Moderate
Anemia

Severe
Anemia

At the top we see, **Healthy "Normal" Red Blood Cells**: These cells are bright red, the center portion, which is the thinnest part of the cell is normally the same color as the rest of the cell. While some red blood cells might be slightly "lighter" than others, most are still entirely normal. The red blood cell is basically round, but may look elliptical when seen on its side.

In **Mild to Moderate Anemia:** Here the red blood cells are more or less deficient in the red dye hemoglobin so that the entire cell looks lighter, almost pink (hypochromic), and they may or may not be smaller (microcytic) than the normal red blood cell, depending on the degree of anemia.

In **Severe Anemia**: These red cell is almost pink, not at all bright red. The red blood cells are now much smaller (*microcytic*) and there are less in total number. In some cells the centers may even be clear which makes them *severely hypochromic* red blood cells.

Figure 1

Bone marrow testing is rarely done and usually only when the diagnosis is in doubt after all other tests have been performed. It is performed in the doctor's office under local anesthesia, and the results usually are available in 2 to 3 days.

Summary of Abnormal Laboratory Finding In Iron Deficiency Anemia				
Finding	**Normal**	**Mild Anemia**	**Moderate Anemia**	**Severe Anemia**
Hemoglobin	13 to 15	10 to 12	37873.0	Below 9
Hematocrit	>35%	30% - 34%	30% - 25%	Below 25%
Peripheral Red Blood Smear	Normal	Mild microcytosis	Microcytosis, anisocytosis, poikilocytosis	
Mean Corpuscular Volume (MCV)	80–100 fL	No change or minimal decrease	Mild to moderate decrease can remain in the normal range even with significant anemia	
Mean Corpuscular Hemoglobin (MCH)	26–34 pg	Decreased MCH with iron deficiency anemia		
Mean Corpuscular Hemoglobin Concentration (MCHC)	31–35 g/dL	Decreased MCHC with iron deficiency anemia		
Ferritin	Above 30 mg/L: Males 16–300 µg/L Females 4–161 µg/L	30µg to 15 µg/L		Below 15 µg/L
Total Iron Binding Capacity (TIBC)	250-460 µg/dl (45-82 µmol/L)	Significantly greater than 460 µg/dl		
RBC Distribution Width (RDW)	Values generally below 15	Elevated greater than 15		

Table 3

Can Other Serious Medical Problems Look Like IDA?

There are other types of anemias and there are other causes of microcytic anemia. These include anemias caused by certain chronic diseases, thalassemia[10], and less commonly a condition called sideroblastic anemia. The anemias caused by chronic diseases are generally characterized by normal or increased iron stores in the liver and bone marrow, and a normal or elevated ferritin level. The TIBC is either normal or low. Thalassemia characteristically produces a greater degree of microcytosis (small red blood cells) for any given level of anemia than does iron deficiency. Red blood cells also become abnormal earlier than in IDA and generally show more target cells at all stages.

Other conditions that can produce microcytic anemia are chronic infections or inflammations, lead poisoning, cancer, liver disease and chronic kidney failure. All of these can be distinguished from IDA when the symptoms caused by these conditions are recognized and because even though serum iron and TIBC are reduced, there is usually a normal or increased serum ferritin, along with normal or increased bone marrow iron stores. During the process of making the diagnosis of IDA, all other conditions must also be eliminated.

Conditions such as rheumatoid arthritis, certain connective tissue disorders, and certain types of injury can also be confused with mild IDA. When anemia occurs with these conditions it is usually directly related to their occurrence. In all cases of IDA should first be ruled out, since it is the most common from of anemia.

Finding The Reason For The IDA

Finding the exact reason for the iron loss is essential not only to the diagnosis of IDA, but also for treating the underlying problem that is causing it. This is especially true when the cause is chronic blood loss. Signs of abnormal bleeding must be sought, and the area of bleeding evaluated to rule out malignancy, ulcer disease, or other treatable causes. It is inappropriate to treat IDA without making sure that there is no serious condition underlying it.

Because of the nature of iron balance in infants, adolescents, and pregnant women it is generally unnecessary to perform extensive evaluations to find the cause of their IDA in most instances, unless other symptoms are present. A trial with iron by diet or supplementation is usually sufficient. However, any abnormality among men or postmenopausal women necessitates prompt and thorough investigation. If there is not a good response to treatment with iron, then a more careful evaluation looking for a cause of the anemia must be initiated.

Chapter 2

Treatment of Iron Deficiency Anemia

IDA should always be treated and reversed. The level of treatment however usually depends on the severity of the condition. In the mildest cases diet alone is all that is necessary, in moderate to moderate severe anemia, diet with medication or supplementation is indicated. In the very worst cases, blood transfusion may be necessary.

How Is IDA Best Treated?

It would seem at first that this would appear to be a straight forward question which would likely have a straight forward and simple answer, but this is not so. It seems that there are really two sets of answers, two camps as one would have it that are often diametrically opposed to each other. Both would agree that giving more iron is the best treatment, but it is how this iron is to be given that in the end sets the two groups apart from each other.

On one side are those individuals who suggest and strongly believe in a nutritional-dietary approach for the prevention and treatment of IDA. On the other side are those individuals who believe in a strictly medical approach for prevention and treatment of IDA. Clearly both sides present their pros and cons and in some circles rail at each other providing a host of reasons why their approach is right and the other side is wrong, and why only their view should be accepted.

The Conventional Medical Approach

The main argument of those individuals who suggest a strictly conventional medical approach is that not only is there a paucity of reliable information regarding diet and nutritional treatment, but also the available information is confusing, frustrating and rarely can be religiously followed. Hence medications, they say are better, since medications can usually be taken regularly and with little risk and the results are generally more reliable and consistent. They often decry supplements as being inconsistent, unreliable, confusing and costly. They often also throw out the argument that even though most people think vitamins and nutritional supplements are safe because they are "natural," that this is not really true. They may even add that it may have once been true, when nutrients were consumed only in their natural form as food, but not once they are put into pill form.

Another favorite argument is against mega (large) doses of vitamins and minerals suggesting that this can be dangerous and that people can ultimately take such large doses that they become poisoned. To conflict with this they argue that if you take these large doses you might well be disturbing your own internal vitamin-mineral balance hence creating long term health problems.

While vitamins-mineral supplements are the more favorite topic of this group certain members also criticize the so-called "therapeutic dietary" approach. While they may admit that the risk of overdose is less likely, they will frequently raise the argument that severe restrictions can ultimately lead to deficiencies of various kinds and they are often quick to add that most of the "fad" dietary approaches to various illnesses have not been systematically studied in human beings, and that proof of their effectiveness has not been established. To this they add that "more research is needed to evaluate the value of these diets in human studies."

The Proponents of Diet and Nutritional Therapeutic Supplements

The non-medical approach group, usually thought of as the "health food" devotee, are often heard to put forth arguments that diet is a more natural way of treating IDA. Many even suggest that the argument about supplements is a non argument for no matter what the medical proponent say all they have to offer is a different brand of supplements to be used to treat anemia. Some might even add that the only difference is that their supplements are usually either prescription medications or over-the-counter single source supplements. In many cases they may even turn the medical profession's arguments against supplements against the medical profession saying that there is little or no difference except for the money for these supplement goes back to the medical establishment. The basic argument of the health food devote is that "medicine is bad, food is good" holds up no matter whether one uses iron from a pharmacy or from a health food store. Many supplement proponents quickly add that the once the same iron found in supplements is made into a medication its cost goes up greatly.

Making Sense Of Both Positions

In the end, both positions are simply personal opinions. While it may be true dietary approaches may need more research and work to prove their value, it is also true that the medical side cannot really show that their approach is much better. Ultimately we can look at it the situation in the following way, "pick which method you feel most comfortable with and do that." Whether you take a pill, swallow a supplement or do it with diet alone, makes little difference as long as it works and anemia is either prevented or reversed." Both groups present good points and bad points, but neither have completely persuasive arguments. Hence, pick which way feels best to you and do that.

It is our goal in this booklet to try our best to make sense out of a dietary approach. If however, you have severe anemia which might take months to treat with diet alone, then be smart use supplements to help speed up the process. Our first choice is amino acid chelated iron, after that we really do not believe that there is any significant difference between one or another type of supplements, prescription or non-prescription over-the-counter medications.

Our main consideration is to instruct our readers to avoid "true believers" those who claim that there is one an only one diet or supplement that will solve all problems. This is rarely true and usually portends a con artist who is pushing his or her product which is usually many times more expensive than it needs to be. In this work we will only provide for you commonly used dietary approaches that can be modified for personal needs, likes and dislikes. Use food as your basic prevention and treatment of mild anemia, supplements or medications only if moderate or severe anemia along with iron rich foods.

Mild IDA Can Be Treated as Follows:

- A careful selection of foods high in iron (See Chapter 3 and Appendices, below) to insure not only high daily intake of iron but a small excess of iron to refill deficient iron stores within the body.

- Add vitamin C to your diet especially when you are eating non-heme iron foods or supplements. Good food sources of vitamin C are listed below (See complete list Appendix D):
  - Oranges and orange juice
  - Lemons and lemon juice
  - Grapefruit
  - Tomatoes and potatoes
  - Broccoli
  - Strawberries
  - Kiwi fruit

- ‣ Bell peppers
- ‣ Hot peppers
- ‣ Green beans
- ‣ Greens

Moderate Anemia Can Be Treated As Follows:

- An iron-rich diet to insure high daily intake if iron an excess of iron to refill deficient iron stores within the body.

- Ferrous sulfate, ferrous fumerate or ferrous gluconate 325 mg taken one to two times a day. The total amount used will likely depend on:
  - ‣ The stage of the iron deficiency (See Tables 2 and 3)
  - ‣ How iron is tolerated, depending on the presence of side effects such as constipation, diarrhea abdominal pain, etc.
  - ‣ Typical each prescribed tablet should betaken after a meal or at bedtime.

Severe Anemia Can Be Treated As Follows:

- An iron-rich diet to insure high daily intake of iron to refill deficient iron stores in the body.

- Ferrous sulfate or ferrous fumerate or ferrous gluconate 325 mg taken three to four times per day. The total amount used will likely depend on:

  - ‣ The level of iron deficiency (See Tables 2 and 3)
  - ‣ How iron is tolerated, depending on presence of side effects such as constipation, diarrhea, abdominal pain, etc.
  - ‣ Typical each prescribed tablet should be taken after a meal or at bedtime.

- On occasion when hemoglobin levels are seriously low, the heart is particularly vulnerable. In this situation either a blood transfusion or injectable iron may be needed to treat severe anemia. Other than based on severe anemia where heart failure is a potential, the use of injectable iron is generally reserved for individuals who:

  - ‣ Have a poor tolerance to iron in any form
  - ‣ Are noncompliant with oral preparations or
  - ‣ Suffer from a serious malabsorption problem.

Depending on how anemic an individual is, hemoglobin values will generally not respond fully for some 30-45 days after treatment is started. While response to iron will start immediately full resolution often depends on a number of factors (other than iron intake alone) including: 1) the type of iron used (heme versus non heme iron), 2) the preparation used for treatment (ferrous versus amino acid chelated iron), 3) the bioavailability of the iron in the specific preparation, 4) the ability of the digestive system to absorb the iron, red blood cell production, 6) vitamin B12 deficiency, 7) deficiencies or excesses of other vitamins, minerals and essential nutrients that will either enhance or block iron absorption and utilization. Most of these we have already discussed above.

How Do You Know If This Treatment (Diet, Medication With Or Without Supplements) Are Working?

Most people will respond quickly to an iron rich diet and iron supplementation with rapid improvement both in their CBC and their general feelings of well-being. When compliance is poor it may be improved by introducing oral iron slowly and by gradually escalating the dosage along with food. An appropriate response to oral iron (dietary or supplement) is a return of the hemoglobin and hematocrit level to at least half way toward normal within 3 weeks with full return to baseline after 2 months. Iron therapy should then continue for 3–6 months after restoration of normal blood values in order to replenish iron stores.

Failure of response (at any point described above) to iron therapy is usually due to noncompliance, although an occasional person may also absorb iron poorly. Other reasons for failure to respond can include 1) an incorrect diagnosis (anemia of chronic disease, thalassemia), or 2) an ongoing gastrointestinal blood loss that exceeds the rate of absorption or production of new red blood cells. Individuals with moderate to severe IDA should stay on iron supplements for at least 6 months or longer to replenish depleted body iron stores.

Iron deficiency anemia on its own is rarely a life-threatening situation. The most important part of treatment is identification of the cause, especially any source of blood loss.

People over 50 years of age with gastrointestinal bleeding should be referral to a specialist for evaluation to rule out a gastrointestinal malignancy.

As many as 25% of people using either ferrous sulfate, gluconate or fumerate may have some nausea, abdominal pain, diarrhea and constipation. If this occurs consult your physician. You may need to change the dose or type of iron you are taking. Stop taking ferrous sulfate, gluconate or fumerate or change to an amino acid chelated iron. After any gastrointestinal surgery, especially a stomach surgery, your body may absorb less iron than normal. In this case a liquid iron preparation may be helpful. Talk with your doctor and ask him to prescribe liquid iron for you.

When 325 mg of ferrous sulfate is taken 3 times a day this will ultimately provide the body with about 180 mg of iron daily. Of this 180 mg of available iron, only about 10 mg of iron will actually be absorbed, at very best. However, in a very few individuals with severe iron deficiency the amount of iron which is ultimately absorbed may exceed this amount. In such situations the body may, to a very limited degree, actually be able to increase its ability to absorb iron. Remember, this only happens in individuals suffering a *severe iron deficiency* problem.

For prevention, we generally suggest to our patients to go to their local health food store and buy a good (not necessarily the most expensive) multivitamin with iron. For the best results make sure that the iron is either amino acid chelated iron or colloidal iron (again, the cost of the preparation generally has little to do with its effectiveness, so you do not have to buy the most expensive preparation). We have them take this preparation for a while and than at about 6 to 8 weeks we have them return to see how they are doing. If IDA was present to begin with we will normally retest at this time. This often also depends on how our patients feel, and a cursory evaluation to assess any symptoms that may persist from the anemia.

Is Too Much Iron a Problem?

About one million people in the United States may be affected by iron overload due to a condition called *hemochromatosis*. Hemochromatosis is a genetic condition characterized by excessive iron absorption, excessive tissue iron stores, and a potential for tissue injury caused by excessive iron in the tissues. It does not happen to people who do not have the genetic dysfunction that makes it happen. If this condition goes undetected or untreated, iron overload may eventually result in the onset of physical problems including cirrhosis of the liver, liver tumors (hepatomas), diabetes, heart problems, arthritis or other joint problems, or reduced functioning of the pituitary gland and atrophy of testes or ovaries). This most commonly occurs in genetically susceptible people between ages 40 to 60 years of age.

The degree and severity of the symptoms of iron overload generally appears to depend on the amount of absorbable iron in the diet, and physiological blood loss from the body (e.g., menstruation). Transferrin saturation test is the recommended screening test for hemochromatosis. An elevated transferrin saturation test (TIBC) can suggest hemochromatosis. Preventing or treating the clinical signs of hemochromatosis involves repeated blood removal to remove excess iron from the individual's body.

Can You Take Too Much Iron Medication or Supplement?

Yes! Treating iron deficiency is one thing but over-treating (taking therapeutic dosages past the time that the deficiency has been resolved) or taking dosages greater than the usual therapeutic dosage, even for short periods of time, can result in iron toxicity or iron poisoning. This can happen either by accident or very occasionally on purpose. Neither is appropriate.

What Are the Symptoms of Iron Toxicity or Iron Poisoning?

Early or Mild Symptoms (will develop the following symptoms within 6 hours of overdose):

- Vomiting with or without nausea
- Explosive diarrhea
- Irritability
- Abdominal pain
- Rapid breathing
- Rapid heart beat
- Low blood pressure
- Greyish color to the skin

Later or More Severe Exposure:

- Bleeding from the bowels (bright red blood or back stools)
- Seizures
- Lethergy (feeling tired or lethargic, foggy, difficult to think, dopey, or stuporous)
- Coma

In the more severe cases the above symptoms, if not treated immediately, will within 10 to 14 hours appear to clear up and get better, however, this does not mean that the individual is out of the woods for within the next 12 to 48 hours the exposed individual may gradually become disorientated, restless, lethargic, develop convulsions, then coma, shock and death can follow, if not treated effectively as soon as is possible.

Late Consequences

If the person survives the initial symptoms and problems, within 2 to 5 weeks later complications can occur. On of the most important symptoms is acute bowel obstruction.

How Much Iron Would Actually Be An Over-Dosage?

In children, especially infants, over-dosage can be lethal. It is not unusual for young children to get into their mother's iron pills and ultimately over-dose and even die. It is essential if you have young children living in your home that iron be kept as far as possible out of the reach of young children. The best place is under lock and key.

The lethal dose in children can be as little as 130 mg total dosage of ferrous or ferric iron in young children. (See Table 4.)

As A Rule of Thumb In Children:

Poisoning In Children	
Mild poisoning can occur after only	10 iron tablets
Moderate poisoning	20 iron tablets
Severe poisoning	greater than 20 iron tablets

Table 4

If you or your child over-doses on iron **** Any Dosage **** call your doctor or go to the nearest local emergency room. Bring the bottle with you so that the doctors can see exactly what was taken. Remember make sure that your children cannot get into your iron pills, put them in a safe place or lock them up.

This is one reason why treatment of IDA should always be undertaken under the supervision of a licenced and experienced physician.

Summary

If You Presently Suffer From IDA:

1. **What Should I Do?**

- If you think you are at risk for IDA, go to your doctor and have a screening blood test for anemia performed.
- If you are pregnant, participate in your prenatal care, and take the iron tablets and prenatal vitamins prescribed for you by your doctor.
- Continue to take your prenatal vitamins and iron, if you are breast feeding.
- Eat a well-balanced diet to maintain your iron balance.

What Should I Not Do?

- Do not over exert yourself while you are anemic, avoid overexertion of any kind.

You Should Talk With Your Doctor Right Away If Any Of The Following Occur:

- If you experience severe fatigue, dizziness, chest pain, irregular heart beat, rapid pulse, shortness of breath or any difficulty breathing. Call your doctor immediately.

- If you have bleeding from the bowels or excessive menstrual bleeding or if any existing bleeding increases. Call your doctor *immediately*.

- If you have abdominal pain from the iron supplements try the following, and if these suggestions do not work, stop taking the iron and speak with your doctor:
  - ▸ Take your iron supplements with food.
  - ▸ Lower the dosage of the iron you are taking for a while and see if this helps
  - ▸ Changing to a different iron formulation. Generally we recommend taking *Amino Acid Chelated Iron* as this preparation is much less likely to cause abdominal pain or discomfort.

(This Page Is Purposefully Left Blank For You To Use To Take Notes)

Chapter 3

Preventing and Treating Iron Deficiency Anemia

Through Your Diet

A Simple Strategy for Prevention and Treatment of IDA

I. Diet High in Iron

The best prevention against IDA is a good healthy balanced diet made up primarily of whole foods along with good healthy food habits.

In the section below we will provide a number of lists of foods which are iron rich. We will also give you a sense of foods which will interfere with and undermine iron absorption as well as lists of foods that will enhance iron absorption. Using these lists we will provide you with a sample menu which is both iron rich and chosen to increase enhancing factors and decrease interfering factors. Using these lists and the sample menu you can now create a healthy iron rich diet based on your own likes and dislikes.

Start by making yourself aware of the Food Pyramid concept of a healthy diet and divide the following choices up into three regular meals each day or four smaller meals each day. Do not skip meals. (See Figure 2.)

Next follow the basic plan listed below:

A) **MEAT - PROTEIN GROUP**: *Two to three - 4 ounces - servings a day.*

Meat, fish and foul should be weighed raw, all fat and bone should be removed before cooking. Most supermarkets will cut and package meats in 4 ounce, boneless, skinless and fat trimmed portions ready for the freezer. Another hint is to have your butcher put wax paper between each slice so that you can separate each slice of meat and package them individually before freezing.

You may select your protein from beef (lean cuts such as round, flank, chuck, T-bone), lamb, pork and veal are all reasonably good sources of heme iron (See Appendix A). The next highest available resource of iron can be found in sea foods especially clams, crab, oysters, octopus, shrimp, fresh white tuna or packed in water, canned sardines, mussels, flounder, cod, halibut and pink salmon. While other sea foods are commonly available, such as yellowtail, bass, white fish, haddock, red snapper, shad, trout, orange roughy, catfish, mackerel, lobster, crayfish, abalone, scallops they appear to generally have lower levels of iron than those listed above and therefore should be eaten only when the above are not available or you have not acquired a taste to utilize them.

In regard to poultry, once again organ meats, especially chicken and turkey liver are listed as the highest resource for available heme iron from poultry. Duck and other wild game meats are also relatively high in iron. Of the domesticated poultry the dark meats of chicken and turkey are highest, however chicken and turkey breast (especially if you suffer from elevated cholesterol or are trying to watch your weight, are also reasonably good resources for iron.

Game meats, if you can afford them and have the taste for them are also reasonably good sources of iron. They are also generally much lower in total fat and cholesterol than domesticated meats. (See Appendix A Heme Iron Rich Foods for suggestions.)

While egg yolks are one of the best source of iron, if you are a vegetarian and do eat eggs, then egg white (either from a separated egg or as egg replacer from the market) can be used as a protein as well. Egg whites are lower in iron as most of the iron in eggs is located within the yolk portion of the egg. If you are a "vegan" vegetarian or do not wish to have animal protein you can substitute 4 oz. portions of defatted soy protein, such as Tofu, (cooked curd or mature seeds) or you can use an approved protein shake. Vegetarians can avoid meat products entirely see our section on Vegetarian Diet and Meal Plans, later on in this section.

FOR MODERATE, MODERATELY SEVERE OR SEVERE IDA:

If you are not suffering from high cholesterol nor existing heart disease add portions of the following foods to your diet as often as possible. If you are committed to treating IDA with diet alone then consider daily or at least periodic use of organ meats, especially liver. As is made clear in Appendix A, Heme High Iron Foods, organ meats are often the richest source of iron of all meats. If you are not into organ meats, then red meats are next especially round steak (top and bottom), ground round, hamburger meats, Salisbury steak, chuck, Porterhouse, shoulder blade, rump roast, T-Bone steak and rib and pot roast. In all cases, watch the fat on the meats you eat. If you eat pork then consider the tenderloin, loin chop, sirloin and shoulder butt as well as lean ham as the smartest choices.

If you are cooking it yourself, then by all means cut off all visible fat before you even start cooking your meats. If you do not cook your own meats then cut off all visible fat before you start eating. No reason to raise your cholesterol while you are solving your anemia problem. As we suggested above game meats and fish have less problematic fat content if you need to watch your intake of fats for any reason.

THE FOLLOWING MEATS SHOULD BE EATEN IN MODERATION:

If you have a problem with your cholesterol or are over-weight the following foods should be eaten in moderation: all liver meats, herring, ribs, and other fattier cuts of meat.

B) **BREAD/GRAIN GROUP**: *AT LEAST two to three servings a day.*

Cereals contain some of the highest levels of iron of any non-heme foods. In Appendix B, we have listed a large number of cereals that contain relatively high iron contents. As we have already stated above cereals have two major problems with using them solely as major part of obtaining dietary iron 1) phytates, which are high in grains, can reduce iron absorption and uptake. 2) Cereals are usually eaten with milk, and milk is high in calcium, and calcium also can reduce uptake and absorption of iron into the body. In addition most available cereals have been first refined, and then processed foods with large amounts of refined sugars being added to make them taste good and get you addicted to them. We strongly suggest that cereal should not be made the mainstay of your dietary resource for obtaining iron. Another suggestion you might consider is that it is better to use soy milk instead of cow's milk with cereal since it does not as high a calcium content. You can also substitute water or apple juice either full strength or diluted for cow's milk when cooking. This is especially helpful when you wish to sweeten your cereal. Finally, if weight is not an issue molasses or brown sugar can be added to your cereals to increase the total amount of available iron.

Breads and other sources of grains: (One serving equals one slice or portion) including Melba Toast, Rye Crisp, Brown Rice cake, Brown Rice-Millet cakes, Brown Rice-Buckwheat cakes, Whole Wheat cakes or low calorie bread sticks by Keebler. One slice of any 30 to 60 calorie whole grain breads is healthier and will help you reduce overall starchy carbohydrates and maintain your weight better. You may also have ½ cup of cooked wild rice (again 30-60 calories per ½ cup of cooked wild rice). Wasa Golden Rye or Multigrain crackers can also be used. Read labels to evaluate total iron content (see our section on Reading Labels below and see Appendix B for additional suggestions).

THE FOLLOWING SHOULD BE AVOIDED:

Cookies, cakes, donuts, bagels, breads baked with white flours, sugar or fats such as butter, lard, Crisco™ or other shortening products. These are all empty calorie foods and provide little real nutrition. Even if they are high in iron or not they are not good, healthy nutrition. They should generally be avoided unless you have no other choice for a specific meal or snack. Whole grain breads and cereals are loaded with nutrition, essential vitamins, minerals and other nutrients and are often higher in iron in any event.

C) **FRUIT GROUP**: *AT LEAST two to four servings a day.*

Since vitamin C helps increase absorption and uptake of iron, having a citrus fruit or food high in vitamin C (see Appendix C) can improve your response to the high iron foods you eat on a daily basis. As you may well notice from Appendix B, Non-Heme High Iron Foods, fruits, generally do not have a great deal of iron. There are a few exceptions to this rule. For example, dried peaches, apricots, raisins, prunes, watermelon, figs and dates have moderate amounts of iron.

No size limits on servings (larger or small portions are okay, also don't forget, the juices of the following fruits are often an excellent source of vitamin C as they are concentrated): lemons, oranges, tangerines, grapefruit, apples, apricots, guava, nectarines, peaches, pears, plums, banana, cantaloupe, honeydew or casaba melon are all okay as are any berries including strawberries, raspberries, boysenberries or blueberries, grapes, pineapples and watermelon.

AVOID THE FOLLOWING FRUITS IF YOU ARE ON A WEIGHT LOSS DIET OR ARE TRYING TO CONTROL YOUR WEIGHT, *AS THEY ARE HIGH IN CALORIES:*

Grapes, pineapples, watermelon, dates, figs, mango, raisins are higher in calories and, if weight loss is desired, should be eaten only in moderation and in small amounts.

D) **COMPLEX CARBOHYDRATE - VEGETABLE GROUP**:

You should have *AT LEAST three to five 1 cup each serving* of vegetables each day. The iron in vegetables belongs to the non-heme sources of iron. Generally non-heme sources of iron are less well absorbed and taken up by the body than heme sources of iron.

Adding vitamins C, A, D and riboflavin (see Appendices D, E, F and G for specific foods) to your diet will help increase uptake and utilization of iron more. Therefore in order to maximize uptake and absorption of iron make sure that each meal contains a balance of iron along with foods high in vitamin C, A, D and riboflavin (vitamin B2) as best as you can.

Vegetables are unique in that they can be eaten raw, lightly steamed, cooked alone or combined. Vegetables are considered "free" foods and large quantities may be eaten as part of meals or as a snack between meals. Not only are vegetables helpful in satisfying hunger, they are also high in vitamins, minerals, enzymes and fiber.

YOU MAY EAT *ALL YOU WANT* OF THE FOLLOWING VEGETABLES. THE FOLLOWING VEGETABLES ARE CONSIDERED TO BE FREE FOODS:

Those vegetables highest in iron (listed alphabetically) are: asparagus, beans of all type (especially baked beans, lentils, navy, pinto, red,), broccoli, collard greens, kale, kelp, peas (black-eyed and green split peas), soy bean, most products (tofu), spinach (non-creamed), Swiss chard, potatoes. See Appendix B, Non-Heme Iron Rich Foods for exact amounts of iron available in each of the foods listed above. Although most canned and baked beans contain a large amount of sugar, they are still an excellent source of iron. Try to use dried, reconstituted beans instead whenever possible and especially if you wish to lose or control your weight.

Other vegetables that are healthy to eat, although lower in iron, are: Amaranth, arugula, alfalfa sprouts, bamboo shoots, beans (all types), beets, beet greens, brussels sprouts, bean sprouts, cabbage, cress, cauliflower, celery, chilies (green, pepperoncini, red, yellow - all high in available vitamin C), Chinese mixed vegetables, chop suey vegetables, chrysanthemum leaves, chives, corn (all types), cowpeas, cucumbers, dandelion greens, eggplant, endive, escarole, garlic, ginger, jicama, kohlrabi, leek, lettuce (all types), lotus root, mung beans, mushrooms (all types), mustard greens, okra, onions, parsley, pea pods, peppers (Bell, red, green, sweet, jalapeno - all high in available vitamin C), pickles (all types), pimento, radishes, radicchio, rutabagas, sauerkraut, shallots, soy bean sprouts, green snap beans, string beans, squash (butternut, Italian, summer, winter or zucchini), tomatoes (fresh, cooked, stewed, puree, Italian and Mexican), tomatillo, turnips and watercress.

THE FOLLOWING VEGETABLES ARE BEST EATEN IN MODERATION IF WEIGHT LOSS OR CONTROLLING WEIGHT IS AN ISSUE:

Serving is ½ cup portions, eaten once or twice a week only. Please do eat them they are high in vitamins minerals and other essential nutrients. Beets, carrots, green peas, squash (butternut, Italian, summer, winter), rutabagas, turnips, potatoes, and pumpkin.

E) **NUTS AND SEEDS**: *One or more servings each day.*

Nuts and seeds can be used as ingredients in many recipes, as a snacks during the day or as part of meal in itself or in your cereals.
Almonds, cashews, peanuts (especially peanut butter,), pine nuts, sesame, pumpkin, squash and sunflower seeds.

In the forms section of this book is a form, Daily Meal Planner, which will allow you to create menus for your own meals so that you know what you are going to make for yourself or for your entire family.

II. About Iron Rich Foods

1. Heme Iron Foods

This group is made up primarily of animal meats and meat products.

Eating lean red meats 3 times a week is generally recommended. Red meat is now leaner, and pork is about equal to chicken in its overall fat content. Buffalo, venison, elk and most other game meats are lower in fat than beef, veal, pork or lamb. These lower fat red meats make good food choices and are often over looked. Although they may be more expensive they can often be found in specialty meat markets. If you are trying to reduce fat in your diet, you will also be reducing red meats, which then means that you will probably also be reducing the iron content of your diet.

Generally speaking three 4 ounce portions of lean red meats, poultry and fish are not only a good source of iron but also protein. When this diet is sustained it will help to maintain iron stores and reserves, and refill depletions in the case of IDA. To obtain more protein use tofu or 1 or 2 cups of skim milk on a daily basis. A 3 to 4 ounce piece of meat can generally be based on the size of the back of your hand and should be as thick as your little finger. Using this technique will help you determine the size of your meat portion without having to weigh it.

Red meat is a significant source of iron for menstruating women. The trend in eating less red meat may increase IDA, especially among young children and women of child bearing age.

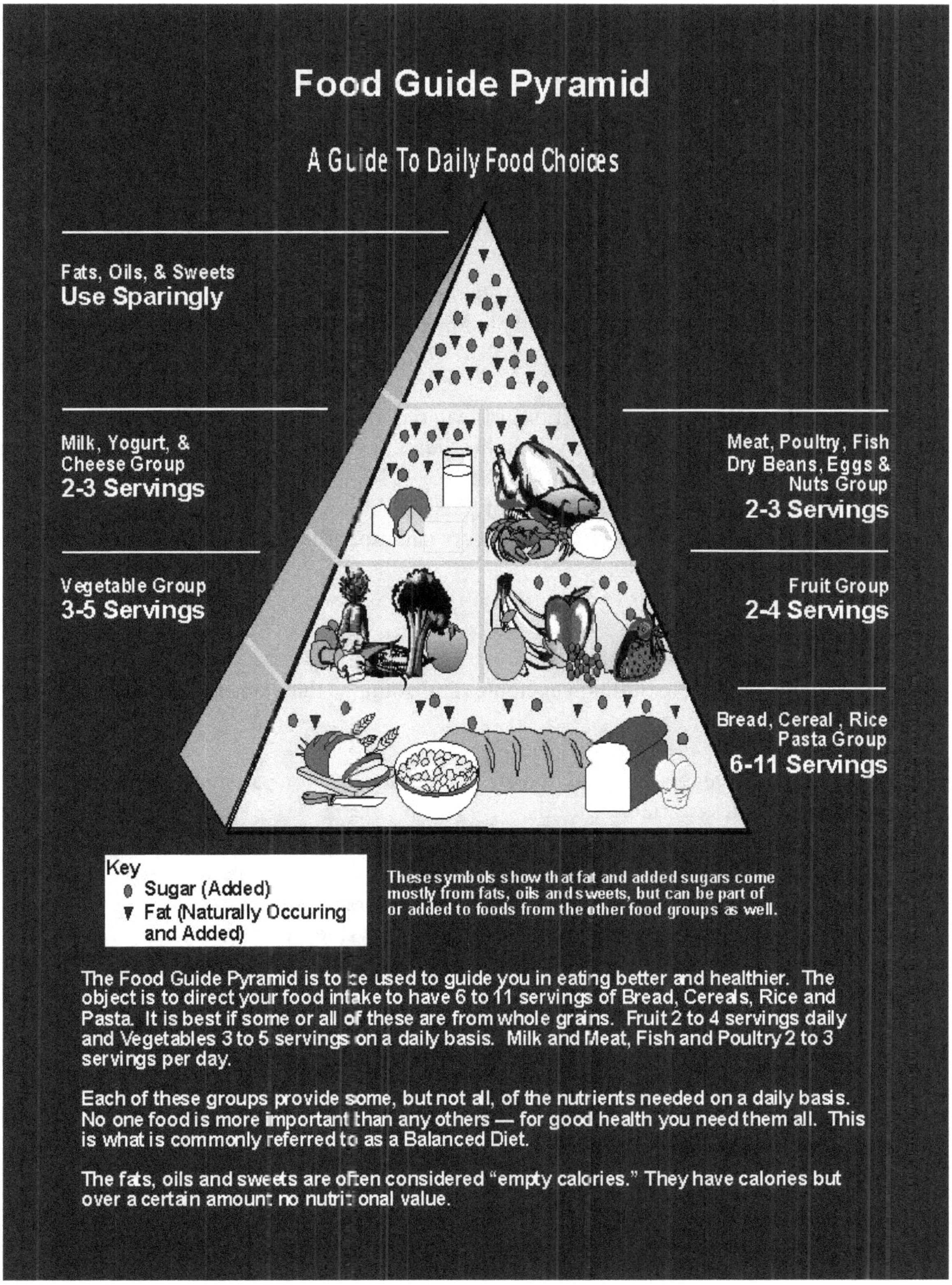

Food Guide Pyramid

A Guide To Daily Food Choices

Fats, Oils, & Sweets
Use Sparingly

Milk, Yogurt, &
Cheese Group
2-3 Servings

Meat, Poultry, Fish
Dry Beans, Eggs &
Nuts Group
2-3 Servings

Vegetable Group
3-5 Servings

Fruit Group
2-4 Servings

Bread, Cereal , Rice
Pasta Group
6-11 Servings

Key
● Sugar (Added)
▼ Fat (Naturally Occuring
and Added)

These symbols show that fat and added sugars come
mostly from fats, oils and sweets, but can be part of
or added to foods from the other food groups as well.

The Food Guide Pyramid is to be used to guide you in eating better and healthier. The object is to direct your food intake to have 6 to 11 servings of Bread, Cereals, Rice and Pasta. It is best if some or all of these are from whole grains. Fruit 2 to 4 servings daily and Vegetables 3 to 5 servings on a daily basis. Milk and Meat, Fish and Poultry 2 to 3 servings per day.

Each of these groups provide some, but not all, of the nutrients needed on a daily basis. No one food is more important than any others — for good health you need them all. This is what is commonly referred to as a Balanced Diet.

The fats, oils and sweets are often considered "empty calories." They have calories but over a certain amount no nutritional value.

Figure 2

III. The Vegetarian Diet

Vegetarians often have normal hemoglobin, but low iron stores (ferritin) in liver, muscles and bone marrow. It is also not unusual that strict non-meat eating vegetarians can develop mild to severe IDA. Iron absorption can, however, often be improved by not only wisely picking iron rich foods but also by adding vitamin C (75 mg per meal equivalent to one 6 oz glass of orange juice) along with an iron supplement (as much as 50 mg per day). ***Iron in the ferrous form within supplements is better absorbed than iron in the ferric form.***

Vegetarian diets, by definition, are low in heme iron. However, iron bioavailability in a vegetarian diet can be increased by careful planning of meals to include other sources of iron and enhancers of iron absorption.

Generally speaking three 4 ounce portions of lean red meats, poultry and fish are not only a good source of iron but also protein. When this diet is sustained it will help to maintain iron stores and reserves, and refill depletions in the case of IDA. To obtain more protein use tofu or 1 or 2 cups of skim milk on a daily basis or nuts and seeds. If you are already a vegetarian, or are starting a vegetarian life style then here are a number of tips to help you prevent IDA:

- Pick more high iron foods to eat with each meal. See our food lists in Appendices A-F at the end of the book.

- Eat a variety of foods including vegetables and grains so that you are not eating the same foods over and over again.

- Get one or more vegetarian cookbooks with recipes that you can make so that you have a relatively endless variety of foods.

- Vary plant-based foods to improve the overall quality the proteins in your diet. For example, if you eat a grain (for example, wheat) which is poor in the essential amino acid lysine with legumes (peas, beans) which are lysine rich you get a high quality of proteins in your diet. Remember that the phytic acid in grains can also interfere with absorption of iron, so do not make them the main part of your diet.

- Egg whites are excellent source of protein and will interfere with nothing.

- While excess dairy (milk, cheese, yogurt, sour cream and butter) can reduce absorption of iron, dairy is essential for its vitamin B12 and zinc so do not eliminate dairy products entirely.

- Use lots of herbs and other natural seasonings to help make your meals tasty.

- Make sure that your diet contains a good amount of foods rich in vitamin C (See our list of vitamin c sources), when ever you eat iron rich foods make sure that your diet also contains rich sources of vitamin C.

Interfering With Iron Absorption

Because vegetarians eat a diet naturally high in fiber and phytates, it can be assumed that they may have more difficulty obtaining iron. Phytates (found in cereals, certain vegetables, roots and nuts, bran and whole grains) can interfere with iron absorption. Oxylates (found in larger amounts in nuts, nut butters, beets, beet greens, teas, strawberries, gelatin, rhubarb, spinach, chocolate and wheat bran) can also interfere with iron absorption from the digestive tract. Fiber which is a major part of the vegetarian diet can also interfere with iron absorption from the digestive tract.

Often as the phytate and fiber content of a specific food or diet increases, so does the iron content. Because of this eating foods which are high in these components will ultimately have much less of an effect on iron absorption than might be expected. The greater overall iron intake compensates for lower bioavailability of this form of iron, that is the greater total iron content of the specific food, the greater the total amount of iron that will ultimately be absorbed.

This is especially true if the food contains more vitamin C or if the foods high in vitamin C are made part of the diet every day. This increased intake of vitamin C appears to reverse the inhibitor effects of phytate in the vegetarian diet. Phytates are also destroyed when nuts and seeds are toasted, by soaking beans before cooking, by sprouting seeds and grains, by adding yeast to breads, and when soybeans are fermented and made into tempeh. Processing of whole grains into refined grains removes large amounts of the phytates, but unfortunately also a significant amount of the iron and natural fiber which originally was in the whole grain.

Iron and The Vegetarian Diet

Only about 20% of available iron in a standard diet comes from meat. Since dairy products are virtually deficient in iron (unless they are enriched), most dietary iron comes from vegetable sources.

The bulk of the available iron in the average diet comes from green leafy vegetables, whole grains, and enriched breads and cereals. Other foods that contain iron can include almonds, avocados, beets, blackstrap molasses, dates, kelp, kidney and lima beans, lentils, millet, parsley, peaches, pears, dried prunes, pumpkins, raisins, rice, wheat bran, sesame seeds and soy beans (see our complete lists in the Appendix sections). On occasion, when somebody cooks in a cast iron pot additional iron may be leached into the diet from these pots.

In order to obtain a maximum amount of iron from the foods eaten vegetarians need to avoid concentrated sources of calcium such as from dairy products. At the same time being careful not to overdose your self on either calcium or zinc supplements. Be sure that these supplements are taken before or after eating foods high in iron.

As we have said repeatedly above, vitamin C enhances the absorption of iron from our diet. For example: when eating brown rice and tofu make sure that they are also served with foods which are high in vitamin C , simply adding tomato sauce and broccoli to your meal can double or even triple your iron absorption.
 Food Combining For The Vegetarian

For a high iron breakfast, try soaking one third cup of seven grain cereal in one half cup of soymilk overnight (throw in a few nuts, dry fruits and seeds). In the morning, add a half cup of water, cook five minutes for a wonderful creamy cereal which is high in iron as well as taste.

The iron in non-meat foods is referred to as non-heme iron. Vegetarians should eat a lot of dark green leafy vegetables (spinach, kale, collard greens dandelion greens), broccoli, asparagus, legumes (lima beans, soybeans, dried beans and peas, kidney beans), yeast leavened whole grain breads (wheat, millet, oats), brown rice, seeds and nuts (sesame, almonds and Brazil nuts), dried fruits (prunes, raisins, apricots), iron-enriched pasta, rice, cereal and textured meat proteins which are high in iron. Unfortunately, the iron in these foods is not as easily and completely absorbed as the iron in meat.

Foods rich in vitamin C (papaya, orange, cantaloupe, broccoli, Brussel sprouts, raw green peppers, grapefruit, strawberries, etc.) can be helpful in improving iron absorption. Remember, sunlight and heat destroy vitamin C so vegetables should be picked as soon as they are ripe and kept in a dark cool place until they are eaten and this should be as soon as is possible after they are picked.

Remember, avoid excessive dairy or dairy products which can block the absorption of iron and lead to iron deficiency. While these foods are high in proteins, they are also low iron. There are soy beverages which have sizable amounts of available iron (also iron fortified infant soy formulas) that you could drink. Look for one to compliment your vegetarian diet.

IV. Tips For Both Vegetarians and Meat Eaters

- No dairy (especially cheese) in the same meal as meats. Remember, calcium blocks the absorption and uptake of the heme iron.

- Have cereal with raisins, and use vitamin D enriched soy milk, instead of cow's milk.

- Use mayonnaise (preferable from soy or canola oil) instead of cheese on hamburgers or sandwich meats.

- Eat more whole foods and avoid as much as possible processed and refined foods as they have considerably less overall nutritional value.

- Add high energy non-heme foods to your diet, for example snack on raisins, dried apricots, figs, prunes, and peaches. Put them in your cereals in the morning.
- Have a citrus fruit or other high vitamin C food along with your heme iron rich meat textured soy or vegetable protein. It can be used as an appetizer or desert, or as a main ingredient or dish within the meal.

- Add foods high in riboflavin, vitamin A and vitamin D periodically to your meals. This can be done. Depending on the food, as a main course, appetizer, ingredient or desert.

- Use our dietary suggestions to pick lower calorie, nutritionally dense foods so that you can easily maintain or even lose weight.

V. Problems and Questions

What About Iron Supplements?

If you are not iron deficient then you do not need to supplement. If you are iron deficient then taking a good supplement either a ferrous iron or better still, an amino acid-chelated iron you can increase your iron absorption. Amino acid chelated iron supplements can increase absorption by 1½ time to 15 times over ferrous or ferric iron.

What About Constipation?

Iron supplements (both ferrous and ferric types, much less likely with amino acid chelated iron) can cause constipation and dark or black stools. To cut down on this side effect make sure that you eat plenty fiber (12 grams per 1,000 calories is usually sufficient) and make sure that you drink plenty water, 8 to 10, 8 ounce glasses of water each day. If these do not work and you cannot switch to an amino acid chelated iron preparation then discuss using a laxative with your doctor.

What About Fortified Foods?

In the course of reading this book you will notice that we believe very strongly in whole organic food diet. Most *fortified* foods are ultimately refined and processed foods and are generally, in our estimation much less healthy for you. If you choose to eat refined and processed foods then look for foods that are fortified, that is have iron added to them. Remember when foods are fortified generally in most cases non-heme, or elemental iron has been added to it. This means that the absorption of this iron is going to be in the 1% to 10% range. In other words no matter how much iron has been added to the specific food you will only be getting between 1% and 10% of it. Therefore if 15 mg has been added to a specific food to fortify it, you will only be able to absorb at very most 1.5 mg of this iron. For this reason foods which have been fortified are usually poor choices overall (they are refined or processed foods + non-heme iron).

Summary

It is important to make sure that your overall diet is a good healthy balanced diet, eat plenty of vegetables and not just the green vegetables (such as salads, or spinach, which by the way has too much oxylates and can in the end block the absorption of iron). Keep the red meat levels down (avoid hardening of the arteries). Chicken, fish and soy proteins are okay. Use the Heme and Non-heme High Iron Food lists Appendices A and B. We also suggest using Appendices D, E, F, and G to support your iron rich diet.

Chapter 4

Reading Labels

1. **Nutritional Facts**
   This box enables you to quickly determine how much of your daily nutrient requirements will be met by eating this specific food. (See Figure 3)

2. **Serving Sizes**
   The servings are meant to standardize the amount of food eaten from item to item and person to person. All the information that follows is based on these amounts. If you eat more or less you should adjust the nutrient amounts.

3. **Calories From Fat**
   Knowing the amount of calories created by fat in the specific food can help you to decide which foods to choose. Notice in Figure 3 more than 50% of the calories in this food is from fat. Present recommendations suggest that fat should make up less than 30% of your daily calories. For optimum health the percentage of fat in your diet should be *no more* than 30%. Ideally the best results occur when there is *no more than* 10% to 20% of calories from fat in the diet. Also please notice the label it is ultimately misleading as it implies that there is only 22% fat when in fact it has *22% of what is expected in a 2000 calorie diet.*

4. **% Daily Value**
   This value tells you how much of a nutrient the product provides. Here one serving supplies 2 grams of dietary fiber which is *8% of the recommended daily consumption of 2,000 calorie-per-day diet.* The goal is to eat an average of close to 100% of the daily requirements each nutrient daily. This listing of saturated fat, cholesterol, sodium and sugars reflect the need for consumers to limit these items. The inclusion of dietary fiber, calcium, iron and vitamins A and C reflect the need to get adequate amounts of these. Magnesium, other B vitamins and other essential nutrients are omitted from this specific

example. They may be found on some labels.

Nutrition Facts

Serving Size 1 cup (236g)
Servings Per Container about 5

Amount Per Serving

Calories 230 Calories from Fat 120

	% Daily Value *
Total Fat 13 g	**22%**
Saturated Fat 5g	35%
Cholesterol 30mg	**13%**
Sodium 118 mg	**5%**
Total Carbohydrates 31g	**5%**
Dietary Fiber 2g	8%
Sugars 3g	
Protein 11g	

Vitamin A 20%	•	Vitamin C 0%
Calcium 2%	•	Iron 6%

* Percent Daily Values are based on a 2,000 calorie diet. Your daily values may be higher or lower depending on your calorie needs

	Calories:	2,000	2,500
Total Fat	Less than	65g	80g
Sat Fat	Less than	20g	25g
Cholesterol	Less than	300mg	300mg
Sodium	Less than	2400mg	2400mg
Total Carbohydrate		300g	375g
Dietary Fiber		25g	30g

Calories per gram:
Fat 9 • Carbohydrate 4 • Protein 4

Figure 3

5. In the % Daily Value section, if we look about halfway down we see that there is130 mg of cholesterol. If you are watching your cholesterol you might want to avoid this food.

6. **Amounts Vitamin A, Vitamin C. Calcium and Iron**
In this book, since we are specifically interested in the iron content of the foods we eat this is an important section. As we have stated earlier Vitamin A, Vitamin D (not included here), Calcium and Vitamin C are all important to either increase or decrease the uptake and absorption of iron. All of these values are important to us in choosing the right foods to eat.

In this section the relative amounts of

these nutrients based on the USDA Recommended Dietary Allowance (RDA) are listed. Hence Iron 6%, indicated that this food contains 6% of the total recommended dietary allowance of iron for any one day. This means that for an average woman (11-50 years of age) where the RDA for iron is 15 mg, this food would contain 6% (or approximately 0.9 mg, a little less than 1 full mg of iron) of this RDA for iron. Similarly, the same would be true for Vitamins A, C and Calcium. In this example, this specific food contains no vitamin C at all, 20% of the RDA for vitamin A and 2% of the RDA for calcium. This means, based on no other considerations, that this would be a "relatively" good food for a person who wanted to increase their iron intake, get some vitamin A and minimal calcium. On the other hand, it has no vitamin C to help improve iron absorption and uptake. It is an okay food to help you treat your IDA, but there are better choices.

7. The Last Two Sections

These last two sections are only included on larger packages. They show 1) Daily amounts of certain nutrients (Total fat, saturated fat, cholesterol, sodium and fiber) required for good health based on both 2,000 and 2,5000 calorie-per-day diets. 2) Calories per gram of fat, carbohydrate and protein. You can use this information when applicable.

8. Is This Food, a Good Food to Eat?

We discussed its value in relation to iron, but what about its overall value and part of a healthy nutritional program? First of all, to answer this question we must ask you to notice that in this example that more than 50% of the calories in this food are from fat. This food also has 31 grams of carbohydrate, 3 grams of which are sugar. We are given no clear idea of how many calories this adds until we look down at the very bottom where we see that fat has 9 calories per gram, proteins and carbohydrates have 4 calories per each gram.

We can now see that the 31 grams of carbohydrates represent 124 calories. Of this 124 calories, there are 3 grams of sugar listed. Three grams x 4 calories per gram equals 12 calories are from this sugar. Since this food does not appear to be a natural fresh food, we might conclude that this sugar is a simple, refined, carbohydrate. Now if we add the total calories from fat 120, to the total from the simple refined sugar 12 calories, we have a totals 132 calories from the combined fat and sugar. This means that this food, whatever it is, contains 57% of the calories form fat and sugar, both of which are probably of little value to the person who eats this food. This would be a *low-nutritional density food*.

Finally, when we evaluate the type of carbohydrate we only know that this is not a fruit or vegetable since this food contains such a large amount of fat. We also know that only 2 grams of this food is fiber. Therefore, we are left with 31 grams of carbohydrate, minus 3 grams of sugar. All of the rest of this food could be starch or grain. Since it is more than likely a processed or refined food, it is likely that any grain in it is processed white flour and hence has little nutritive value. If it is starch, then we have 26 grams (104 calories) more of empty non-nutritive food. This increases the total of non-nutritive food to nearly 95%. This is not likely to be a good food as it is composed of 95% *empty calories*.

(This Page Is Purposefully Left Blank For You To Use To Take Notes)

Chapter 5

Special Situations

The Pregnant Woman

Iron deficiency during pregnancy is relatively common. Most women come into pregnancy already deficient in iron stores. This deficiency, as we have discussed above, generally relates to years of poor diet, eating refined and processed foods, menstruation and increased drainage often created during prior pregnancies. During the course of pregnancy existing stores of iron will be divided between mother and baby. The baby usually will have first priority over the mother's needs.

Pregnant women will need as much as 30 milligrams of iron per day. The main reason is because the unborn baby needs iron for development. As a result, it will draw from the mother's iron stores. This can quickly deplete a woman of iron if she is not eating enough iron rich foods

Iron Deficiency During Pregnancy

During the first two trimesters of pregnancy, women suffering from IDA have a twofold increased risk for preterm delivery and a threefold increased risk for delivering a low-birth weight baby. Iron supplementation along with an iron rich diet can decrease the risks of iron-deficiency anemia during pregnancy. There still is a question as to whether all problems created by existing iron deficiency can be entirely reversed if allowed to exist for prolonged periods of time before iron supplementation is started. In other words no woman should allow her self to become iron deficient if she is planning to become pregnant. Early treatment is a much better idea than waiting to see what happens.

During the course of the most normal and healthy pregnancy, blood volume and total red cell production will also rise to meet the mother's needs as her blood volume expands to support the baby. Between the baby's need for iron and the mother's increased need for iron even perfectly normal stores of iron can become significantly reduced. When a woman begins a pregnancy even marginally depleted in iron the needs of pregnancy will further diminish available stores and can cause IDA.

Primary prevention of iron deficiency during pregnancy includes adequate dietary iron intake and iron supplementation.

Most prenatal vitamins are relatively high in calcium because of the increased need for calcium during pregnancy. Therefore it is not a good idea to take prenatal vitamins and iron at the same time. Take your prenatal vitamins in the morning with breakfast and your iron supplements at night just before dinner and make sure that you have a healthy serving of some food or juice which contains lots of vitamin C.

Primary Prevention

- Start oral, low-dose (30 mg/day) supplements of iron at the first prenatal visit.

- Encourage pregnant women to eat iron-rich foods and foods that enhance iron absorption.

- Pregnant women whose diets are low in iron are at additional risk for IDA.

- Pregnant women with low iron diets need to how to optimize their dietary iron intake.

Screening:

- Screen for anemia at the first prenatal care visit. Use the anemia criteria for the specific stage of pregnancy that applies to each woman.

Diagnosis

- Have your doctor confirm a positive anemia screening result by performing a repeat Hemoglobin concentration or Hematocrit test. If the pregnant woman is not ill, a presumptive diagnosis of IDA can be made and treatment begun.

- If Hemoglobin concentration is less than 9.0 g/dL or Hematocrit is less than 27.0%, ask your doctor to refer you to a physician familiar with anemia during pregnancy for further medical evaluation.

Treatment

- Ask your doctor about treating the anemia by prescribing an oral dose of 60-120 mg/day of iron. Pregnant women should take action about correcting iron-deficiency anemia through the use of prescribed medication or iron supplements (amino acid chelated iron) and an iron rich diet.

- The pregnant woman should eat a diet which has an adequate amount of meats (heme based iron) along with leafy vegetables and other non-heme based iron rich foods.

- The pregnant woman should eat at least one vitamin C rich fruit after each iron rich meal in order to enhance the absorption of all available iron.

- It also helps to delay drinking of tea or coffee for a few hours after each iron rich meals in order to avoid inhibiting the absorption of all available iron in the foods which just have been eaten.

- Further evaluation of the anemia by having other tests, including MCV, RDW, and serum ferritin concentration done. If after 4 weeks the anemia does not respond to iron treatment, or if the woman remains anemia for her specific stage of pregnancy has not improved. Also, the above testing may be needed if the hemoglobin concentration has not increased by at least 1g/dL or a hematocrit value of at least 3% increase, despite compliance with an iron supplementation regimen and the absence of acute illness. In women of African, Mediterranean, or Southeast Asian ancestry, mild anemia unresponsive to iron therapy may be due to thalassemia minor or sickle cell trait.

- When hemoglobin concentration or hematocrit does become normal for the stage of pregnancy ask your doctor about decreasing the dose of iron to 30 mg/day.

- During the second or third trimester, if hemoglobin concentration is greater than 15.0 g/dL or hematocrit is greater than 45.0%, a woman should be evaluated for potential pregnancy complications related to poor blood volume expansion.

Postpartum Women

Women at risk for anemia at 4-6 weeks postpartum should once again be screened by their doctor for anemia by using a hemoglobin concentration or hematocrit test. The anemia criteria for nonpregnant women should be used (See Section 1). Risk factors include anemia continued through the third trimester, excessive blood loss during delivery, and a multiple birth. Treatment and follow-up for IDA in postpartum women are the same as for nonpregnant women. If no risk factors for anemia are present, supplemental iron is usually stopped after delivery.

The Breast Feeding (Lactating) Woman

Breastfeeding can lead to *lactation amenorrhea* (a delay in the return of menstruation). This can be beneficial to women with low iron reserves or who suffer from above-average menstrual blood loss. These women are generally at greater risk for iron deficiency. Lactation amenorrhea conserves iron stores in these women even after the iron which is secreted into their breast milk. It can also help to delay future pregnancies. Lactation amenorrhea can last for 18 months or more hence preserving valuable iron supplies for the mother.

Just as with the pregnant woman, the lactating woman must eat a diet which has an adequate amount of meats (heme based iron) along with leafy vegetables and other non-heme based iron foods. She must also eat at least one vitamin C rich fruit after each iron rich meal in order to enhance the absorption of all available iron. In addition she should delay drinking tea or coffee for a few hours after each iron rich meal in order to avoid inhibiting the absorption of all available iron in the foods which have just been eaten.

Anemia in Infants and Children

Iron is especially important for babies and young children. They must have enough iron in their diet since they grow very rapidly. Babies doubling their birth weight in the first six months and continue to grow until adulthood at an accelerated rate. If children do not get enough iron in their diets they are likely to develop IDA which can then cause then to feel tired and may cause difficulty in concentrating. It may also slow down physical and mental development.

Symptoms in Infants And Children

In infants (newborn through 12 months) and preschool children (ages 1-5 years) who suffer from anemia with a hemoglobin of less than 10, iron-deficiency anemia can result in delays in social and motor development as well as behavioral problems. For example, these children may experience reduced attention span, decreased motor activity, decreased social interaction, and poor attention at tasks. These delays and problems can remain past school age (i.e., 5 years) if the iron deficiency is not rapidly reversed. Iron-deficiency anemia can also contribute to lead poisoning in children by increasing the gastrointestinal tract's ability to absorb heavy metals, including lead. Iron-deficiency anemia is often also associated with conditions that can independently affect infant and child development that may need to be taken into account when evaluating and treating IDA. Babies at higher risk can be so as a result of low birth weight, generalized undernutrition, poverty, and high blood level of lead.

I. Infants (Ages 0-12 Months) and Preschool Children (Ages 1-5 Years)

A full term, healthy baby, whose mother was not severely anemic will be born with iron stores which should last for at least 4 months after delivery. If a baby is not receiving a regular daily intake of adequate iron, this supply of iron will gradually be depleted and the baby will ultimately become anemic. Illness or inadequate diet can create anemia even earlier. Currently the best source of dietary iron for infants under the age of one year is mainly from iron fortified formula or breast milk.

Premature babies often have low stores of iron at birth and are highly susceptible to the problems of IDA if not recognized and treated early.

How Do The Symptoms of Anemia Differ In Infants and Very Young Children?

While the symptoms of IDA are not too much different in infants and children from those in adults, there are certain differences which can help parents recognize that their child may be anemic.

- Infants and children may appear to be irritable, "cranky" or difficult. They may cry easier, have a shorter attention span or even be more fussy.

- Children may act and seem to be tired or fatigued easily, as well appear to be weaker than usual.

- They may look pale since their skin is much thinner hence the usual pallor with anemia is seen sooner and appears more profound. The white part of the infant's eyes may appear to have a bluish cast to them.

- They may have a poor appetite and refuse to eat or have no interest in food.

- Iron deficient children may be seen eating dirt or chewing paint chips, ice, and other mineral-containing substances and objects.

- They may experience headaches which are often missed in younger children and recognized only as listlessness, crying, crankiness and behavior problems.

- In most children the anemia never gets severe enough to cause noticeable symptoms.

- In mild to moderately severe IDA children can manifest decreases in attention span, alertness, and learning ability

- In severe IDA, cognitive[11] development can be slowed down and even stopped, in very severe cases.

- Prolonged or severe anemia can cause increased irritability, further decrease of the appetite, slowed growth, a swollen tongue, flattened, spoon-shaped, or brittle nails. There may be irritated sores at the corners of the mouth.

- In very severe cases, children can even go into heart failure.

The most common reason for IDA in children is either a lack of iron in their diet or they are unwilling to eat sufficient iron containing foods. One should never however, ignore the possibility of blood loss from the bowel or a tumor as a possible cause.

If You Are Breast Feeding Your Baby

The intestines of children who are being breast fed are two to three times more efficient at absorbing iron from every source. We encourage breast feeding of infants for the following reasons:

- Breast milk is an excellent first source of iron because the iron in breast milk is easily absorbed by the infant. The main food source for infants under 12 months of age should be breast milk since cow's milk is not a good source of iron. By the time your baby reaches four months of age, they will have used up all of their iron stores. After this, they will become entirely dependent on their diet for all of the iron they will need to make red blood cells and maintain all of their other bodily needs.

- While breast milk is low in iron, it is higher in lactose and contains more vitamin C than cow's milk. Ultimately, this means up to 48% better absorption of the iron that is in breast milk.

- We encourage the exclusive breast feeding of infants (without supplementary liquid, formula, or food) for 4-6 months after birth. Of course, this assumes that the mother is not iron deficient.

- When exclusive breast feeding is stopped, we encourage the use of an additional source of iron (approximately 1 mg/kg per day of iron), preferably from supplementary foods or consult your pediatrician about iron supplementation along with supplementation of other essential vitamins and minerals.

- As with adults the form of the iron ingested and the other foods that are eaten in the same meal, will determine how much iron can be actually absorbed by the digestive system. Once again, the best source of iron is red meats. The iron in red meats is most easily absorbed. Some plant foods, such as beans and lentils, also contain a lot of iron, but the body does not absorb the non-heme iron from plant foods very well.

- Remember that foods high in vitamin C will help your baby absorb more iron from both meat and plant sources. Make sure that you include a high vitamin C food source with every iron rich meal. See the list of high iron and high vitamin C baby foods. You can always make your own combinations from the adult high iron and high vitamin C foods lists.

- When you plan an iron rich red meat meal, do not include peas, beans and lentils in the same meal as they can interfere with absorption of iron. Babies should never be given tea or coffee in any appreciable amount as they too can interfere with the absorption of iron.

- If you are continuing to breast feed your baby even after starting solid foods try to feed the solid foods at different times than when you breast feed so that your baby can absorb as much iron as possible.

- Extra care should be taken with infants on a vegetarian diet to ensure that they receive enough iron from non-meat sources, and a plentiful supply of vitamin C rich foods.

- For infants under12 months, who are not breast fed at all, or who are only partially breast fed, the use of iron-fortified infant formula as a substitute for breast milk is strongly recommend.

- For breast-fed infants who receive insufficient iron from supplementary foods by age 6 months (i.e., less than 1 mg/kg per day), supplemental iron drops, 1 mg/kg per day of iron each day, is suggested.

- For breast-fed infants who were premature or preterm or had a low birth weight, 2-4 mg/kg per day of iron drops (to a maximum of 15 mg/day) starting at 1 month after birth and continuing until 12 months after birth is usually recommend. Once again check with your pediatrician.

Milk and Infant Formulas

- Encourage use of only breast milk or iron-fortified infant formula for any milk-based part of the diet (e.g., in infant cereal) and discourage use of low-iron milks (e.g., cow's milk, goat's milk, and soy milk) until age 12 months. (See Table 4)

- It is suggest that children between the ages of 1year and 5 years old consume no more than 24 oz of cow's milk, goat's milk, or soy milk each day.

Once Your Child Is Eating Solid Foods:

- At age 4-6 months or when the extrusion reflex[12] disappears, it is recommend that infants be introduced to plain, iron-fortified infant cereal (for example Iron Fortified Pablum). Two or more servings per day of iron-fortified infant cereal can meet an infant's requirement for iron at this age.

- By approximately age 6 months, encourage one feeding per day of foods rich in vitamin C (e.g., fruits, vegetables, or juice) to improve iron absorption, preferably with meals.

- It is advisable to introduce pureed meats after age 6 months or when the infant is developmentally ready to consume such food. Once again speak with your pediatrician about when the time is right for your baby.

- Between eight and nine months of age start iron rich foods like liver and red meats. Unfortunately, the quantity of iron rich foods needed to prevent anemia in infants under the age of one, is more than an infant could usually eat. So if your baby continues to take formula make sure that it is an iron-fortified formula.

Iron Absorption In Infants Fed Formula, Cow's Milk and Breast Milk			
Formula /Milk	Iron Content	Bioavailable Iron in %	Total Absorbed Iron
Regular Non-fortified formula[1]	1.5 to 4.8 mg/L	~10 %	0.15-0.48 mg/L
Iron-fortified formula [1,2]	10.0 to 12.8 mg/L	~ 4 %	0.40-0.51 mg/L
Whole cow's milk	0.5 mg/L	~10 %	0.05 mg/L
Breast milk	0.5 mg/L	~50 %	0.25 mg/L
[1] Values are given for commonly marketed infant formulas. [2] Iron-fortified formula contains >=1.0 mg iron for each100 calories of the formula. Most iron-fortified formulas contain approximately 680 kcal/L, which is equivalent to >=6.8 mg iron/L of the formula.			

Table 4

Preventing And Treating Amenia In Children

Preventing and treating IDA in small children can often be quite difficult because of the child's likes and dislikes and food avoidance patterns.

There are some foods which children are usually more willing to eat and can be made a stable part of their diet which can help to both prevent and treat IDA.

The best source of iron in very young children is breast milk (as the iron in breast mild is very easily absorbed by children) or formulas and infant cereals fortified with iron. In older children who are already eating solid foods try Cream of Wheat, Total, Product 19, other iron-fortified cereals, liver and prune juice are also rich iron sources.

For older children you can also make sure that their daily diet has one or more of the following:

Eggs, meats, fish (tuna is often well accepted), chicken, turkey, soybeans, cooked beans, peanut butter, peas, lentils, molasses. See the food lists in Appendices A for additional help with meats.

You can add some of the following: oatmeal, apricots, raisins, spinach, kale, greens, prunes or prune juice. See the food lists in Appendices B-F for additional iron sources.

What Can Be Done To Help With Absorption Of Iron In Children?

Taking vitamin C, or eating foods high in vitamin C (such as orange juice) at the same time as foods high in iron will help the child's body absorb and use the iron. The iron in iron-fortified foods is poorly absorbed, but usually contains enough extra iron to compensate for this. Over-the-counter or prescription multivitamins with iron can help provide a safety net for picky eaters. For young children multivitamins with iron can be given in a liquid form. Mother need only give a few drops each day (dosage is based on age and severity of the anemia. Only under a doctor's care and instructions). The drops can be placed in juice or even directly in the child's food. Ferrous iron drops can turn the child's stool black and may in some situations cause constipation, no matter how they are given.

What Foods Will Block Absorption Of Iron In Children?

Cow's milk, which is the basis of most infant formulas, contains very little iron and very little vitamin C. As a result of this it can interfere with the absorption of any iron, supplemental or dietary, in your baby's diet. If your child drinks too much cow's milk this can actually make his or her anemia worse. Large amounts of cow's milk can cause a child to lose iron through the intestines, and can also make it more difficult for their body to use any iron that is present in the foods they eat. Most toddlers get sufficient calories and calcium from 16-24 ounces of milk daily. No child needs more than 32 ounces of cow's milk a day. *Almost all cases of severe iron deficiency in young children are in those who drink too much milk.*

Secondary Prevention

Even though our body does have natural iron regulatory mechanisms to increase absorption of iron when we are in the process of becoming iron deficient, these mechanisms may be of little value if the diet itself is deficient. Early diagnosis allows for early treatment.

Universal Screening:

- In populations of infants, toddlers and preschool children at high risk for iron-deficiency anemia (e.g., children who are growing rapidly and may have insufficient iron available in their diet, children with rigid likes and dislikes, who avoid iron rich foods, children in low-income families, migrant children, or recently arrived refugee children). It is wise to screen all children for anemia between ages 6 and 12 months, 6 months later, and annually from ages 2 to 5 years.

Selective Screening:

- In populations of infants, toddlers and preschool children who are not at high risk for iron-deficiency anemia, only those children who have known risk factors for IDA need be screened.

- Parents and physicians should consider anemia screening before age 6 months for any preterm infant or low-birth weight infant who is not being fed iron-fortified infant formula.

- During annual physical and examination it is always wise to assess children who are between the ages of 2-5 years for risk factors of iron-deficiency anemia (e.g., a low-iron diet, limited access to food because of poverty or neglect, or special health-care needs). Screen these children if they have any of these risk factors.

- At ages 9-12 months and 6 months later (at ages 15-18 months), assess infants and young children for risk factors for anemia.

The Following Children Should Be Screened for IDA:

- Any preterm or low-birth weight infant

- Any infants who are fed a diet of non-iron-fortified infant formula for greater than 2 months

- Any infants introduced to cow's milk before age 12 months

- Any breast-fed infant who, after age 6 months, does not consume a diet with an adequate amount of iron (i.e., who has received insufficient iron from supplementary foods)

- All children who consume greater than 24 oz of cow's milk on a daily basis

- All children who have special health-care needs (that is, children who use medications that interfere with iron absorption and children who have chronic infection, chronic inflammatory disorders, restricted diets, or extensive blood loss from a wound, an accident, or surgery).

II. IDA in School-Age Children (Ages 5 t0 12 Years) and Adolescent Boys (Ages 12- to less than 18 Years)

If you have a school-aged child or adolescent boy, only those with a history of iron-deficiency anemia, special health-care needs, or low iron intake need be screened for anemia. Age-specific anemia criteria should be used, your pediatrician will know exactly what needs to be done.

Treating School Age Children And Adolescent Boys:

The treatment of iron-deficiency anemia in this group includes a minimum treatment (depending on the severity of the anemia which is usually mild) one 60-mg iron tablet each day for school-age children and two 60-mg iron tablets each day for adolescent boys. Dietary counseling with attention to helping them make regular choices of iron-rich foods is also very important.

Follow-up and laboratory evaluation for school-age children and adolescent boys are basically the same as with infants and preschool children discussed above.

Treatment Of Recognized Anemia In Infants And Young Children:

- Check a positive anemia screening result by having your doctor perform a repeat Hemoglobin concentration or Hematocrit test. If the tests agree and the child is not ill, a presumptive diagnosis of iron-deficiency anemia can be made and treatment begun.

- Your doctor may wish to initiate treatment of presumptive iron-deficiency anemia, even before the laboratory testing has been returned, by prescribing 3 mg/kg per day of iron drops to be administered between meals. The pediatrician should also counsel the parents or guardians about adequate diet to correct the underlying problem of low iron intake.

- Repeat the anemia screening in 4 weeks. An increase in Hemoglobin concentration of greater than or equal to 1 g/dL or in Hematocrit of greater than or equal to 3% confirms the diagnosis of iron-deficiency anemia. If iron-deficiency anemia is confirmed, reinforce dietary counseling, continue iron treatment for 2 more months, then recheck Hemoglobin concentration or Hematocrit. Reassess Hemoglobin concentration or Hematocrit approximately 6 months after successful treatment is completed.

- If after 4 weeks the anemia does not respond to iron treatment despite compliance with the iron supplementation regimen and the absence of acute illness, further evaluate the anemia by using other laboratory tests, including MCV, RDW, and serum ferritin concentration. For example, a serum ferritin concentration of less than or equal to 15 µg/L confirms iron deficiency, and a concentration of greater than 15 µg/L suggests that iron deficiency is not the cause of the anemia.

- **It is important to keep iron tablets out of the reach of children. A large number of young children have died after mistaking iron tablets for sweets.**

It Is Important to Keep Iron Tablets out of the Reach Of Children

---

Adolescent Girls (Females 12- less than 18 Years) and Nonpregnant Women of Childbearing Age

Primary prevention of iron deficiency for adolescent girls and nonpregnant women of childbearing age is through diet. Information about healthy diets, including good sources of iron, is available in Nutrition and Your Health: Dietary Guidelines for Americans (14).

Screening for, diagnosing, and treating iron-deficiency anemia are secondary prevention approaches. Age-specific anemia criteria should be used during screening

III. IDA in Young Girls

Most adolescent and teenage girls and young women do not require iron supplementation, however, it is valuable for parents to encourage them to eat iron-rich foods and foods which can enhance iron absorption. Young women who have low-iron diets are at additional risk for iron-deficiency anemia and parents should work at guiding these young women in optimizing their dietary iron and enhancing food intake by using the guidelines outlined in this book.

IDA in young girls, teens or early twenties, has a number of different causes:

● It is not unusual for young girls who have just started menstruation to become "mildly anemic." The problems are two fold: 1) If the girl is bleeding just enough to mildly drop her hemoglobin level, or 2) She may not be taking in enough iron to cover her new losses.

● Not all young girls are really anemic. This is especially true if the young girl is seen during their menstrual period or immediately after. Their hemoglobin or hematocrit tests may suggest that anemia exists, but if they are retested between menses or 10 days after menstruation, they may be perfectly normal. The slight drop initially seen is usually due to their acute bleeding. The return to normal is based on a good diet with adequate iron stores replenishing the red cells that remain or are newly created. It clearly appears that the time in the menstrual cycle when the blood samples are taken is very important.

● Many young women have low hemoglobin levels and this may be perfectly normal for them. On occasion physicians may forget that diagnostic laboratory testing is generally based on a range of values. Some young girls may normally have hemoglobin values just below what might generally be considered normal and yet actually be "perfectly normal." It is important to remember that one should always make a determination of normal not on what is normal for a lot of people (the general population), but rather what is normal for the specific individual.[13]

● Once again treatment will depend on the severity of the anemia. See the section of Treatment of Amenia.

Screening Young Women For IDA

● Starting in adolescence all nonpregnant women should be screened for anemia every 5-10 years throughout their childbearing years. This is often best done during routine health examinations.

- Annual screening for women who are at increased risk factors for IDA is important. This would include women with heavy menstrual periods or other forms of blood loss, who have low iron intake (iron poor diet) or a previous diagnosis of iron-deficiency anemia.

Diagnosing And Treating Young Non-Pregnant Women

- Confirm a positive anemia screening result by having your doctor perform a repeat Hemoglobin concentration or Hematocrit test. If the adolescent girl or woman is not ill, a presumptive diagnosis of iron-deficiency anemia can be made and treatment begun.

- The usual treatment for adolescent girls and women who have anemia is to prescribe a dose of 60-120 mg of iron to be taken orally each day. These women should also be counseled on how to add iron rich foods into their daily diet.

- If after 4 weeks the anemia does not respond to iron treatment despite compliance with the iron supplementation regimen, and there is no other acute illness to account for the lack of results, then your doctor may want to order additional laboratory tests, including MCV, RDW, and serum ferritin concentration to further evaluate you and your anemia. In women of African, Mediterranean, or Southeast Asian ancestry, mild anemia unresponsive to iron therapy may be due to thalassemia minor or sickle cell trait.

- If the anemia is steadily and suitably resolving, they should then continue iron treatment for at least 2-3 months or more. This will depend on laboratory testing results, and what their doctor feels is appropriate to allow them to return fully to normal and replenish their internal iron supplies.

Men (Males Aged greater than or equal to 18 Years) and Postmenopausal Women

No routine screening for iron deficiency is recommended for men or postmenopausal women. Iron deficiency or anemia detected during routine medical examinations should be fully evaluated for its cause. Men and postmenopausal women usually do not need iron supplements unless they have symptoms of IDA.

Pica

Pica is often classified as an eating disorder which is characterized by cravings for and desire to eat any material that is not generally considered to be food. Individuals who indulge in pica eat laundry starch, dirt or clay, ashes, rubber, crayons, cotton, grass, ice, cigarette butts, soap, twigs, wood, paper, metal, or plaster. Chewing starch, clay, ice or paper is a common symptom of iron deficiency with or without IDA. If it is recognized and the underlying iron deficiency is treated then the pica will stop as the individual's iron levels come up to normal levels. A suggested hemoglobin of 13 to 15 in menstruating women is considered optimal.

Fatigue

Fatigue is one of the most common symptoms of IDA. It can however also be a symptom of a number of other medial and non-medical problems. If you are fatigued, and it has been shown to be caused by IDA, then you should start a treatment program as prescribed by your doctor.

Fatigue is caused in IDA because iron is necessary for the formation of hemoglobin and it is hemoglobin which carries oxygen in red blood cells. When iron levels are low then hemoglobin levels are also low. When this happens a person will often feel tired and lack energy. It may be difficult to do every day tasks due to lack of adequate oxygen delivery to organs and tissues. This is because a red blood cell lives only 120 days. It may take up to 4 months before you feel good once again if you allow yourself to become severely anemic.

Living With IDA

If you have mild IDA the only symptom you might experience is a mild to moderate sense of fatigue. As it progresses the fatigue may also progress causing easy fatigability and some difficulty performing normal daily tasks and activities. The degree and severity of all symptoms may be made worse with acute blood loss. Symptoms may however, be more difficult to recognize when there is a very slow or gradual onset of anemia from either dietary deficiency or minimal gastrointestinal bleeding. In severe cases, especially when there is a more acute loss of blood, some individuals may experience shortness of breath, rapid pulse, irregular heart beat, and even chest pain. If moderately severe to severe iron deficiency occurs over a long period of time other symptoms such as sores in the corners of the mouth, difficulty swallowing, or a tendency for the nails to soften, curl, and sometimes even take on a spoon-like shape, may occur.

(This Page Is Purposefully Left Blank For You To Use To Take Notes)

Appendices

(This Page Is Purposefully Left Blank For You To Use To Take Notes)

Using The Appendices

Instructions For Using Appendices:

1. The following appendices list hundreds of foods, foods high in Iron, Vitamin C, Vitamin A, Vitamin D and Riboflavin (vitamin B2).

2. These list do not contain all of the foods available in the U.S.A. or other parts of the world.

3. The values listed are based on several sources and therefore you may find that certain foods have different values on different lists or may be listed one or more times with different values as the values come from different sources.

4. These lists are provided to you so that you have choices in picking out the best foods for you which are high in iron and high in those nutrients vitamins C, D, A and riboflavin (vitamin B2) which will increase your ability to absorb and take up the iron in your diet.

5. In most cases, the amount of iron listed in each of these lists is based on the amount of iron in 100 grams or approximately 4 ounces (1 cup) of the specific food. If you, for example you chose a food that has 20 mg of iron for each 100 grams of the specific food, and you eat 8 ounces or 2 cups of this food, you will then actually be getting 40 mg of iron from this food. If you should take this same food and reduce the amount you eat, for example you eat only 2 ounces, half of the listed serving, then you would accordingly reduce the total iron available to 10 mg.

(This Page Is Purposefully Left Blank For You To Use To Take Notes)

Appendix A

Heme Foods High In Iron

Food Name	Iron (mg/100grams)
Beef	
Beef Spleen, Raw	44.6
Beef Spleen, Braised	39.4
Calf Liver	18.3
Veal Spleen, Raw	9.3
Beef Lung, Raw	8.0
Beef Heart, Simmered	7.5
Beef Kidney, Raw	7.4
Veal Spleen, Braised	7.4
Beef Kidney, Simmered	7.3
Beef Liver, Raw	6.8
Beef Liver, Braised	6.8
Beef, Top Round, Lean	1 slice = 6.5
Beef, Lean Ground; 10% Fat	6.5
Sirloin, Lean, Broiled	6.2
Beef, Bottom Round, Lean	1 slice = 6.1
Beef Liver, Pan Fried	6.3
Beef, Round Steak Stew Meat	5.5
Salisbury Steak Gravy/Onions	5.4
Hamburger, Lean	5.0
Chuck, Lean	4.9
Rump Roast, Lean (Pot Roasted)	4.9
Porterhouse Steak, Lean	4.9
Veal Liver, Raw	4.8
Blade Steak, Lean	1 steak 4.6

Heme Foods High In Iron

Food Name	Iron (mg/100grams)
T-Bone, Club or Rib Steaks, Lean	4.6
Roast Beef	4.6
Beef Heart, Raw	4.6
Pot Roast, Arm/Blade, Lean	2 slices = 4.1
Short Ribs, Braised	½ lb. = 4.0
Arm Steak, Lean	1 steak 4.0
Beef, Corned	3.9
Beef Shank, Cross Cuts, Choice, Lean	3.8
Beef Chuck, Arm Pot Roast, Choice, Lean	3.8
Beef Chuck, Stewing Beef, Lean, Trim,	3.7
Beef Tenderloin, Choice/Select Lean, Fat, Roasted	3.7
Beef Chuck, Blade Roast, Choice, Lean, Braised	3.6
Beef Tenderloin, Choice, Lean, Fat, Broiled	3.4
Beef Flank, Choice, Lean, Fat, Braised	3.4
Beef Bottom Round, Choice, Lean, Braised	3.4
Beef Steak, Lean, Fried	3.3
Beef Hip, Outside or Bottom Round Steak, Lean, Braised	3.3
Beef Chuck, Arm Pot Roast, Select, Lean and Braised	3.3
Beef Tongue, Simmered	3.2
Beef Chuck, Arm Pot Roast, Lean, Braised	3.2
Beef Short Ribs, Choice, Lean, Braised	3.2
Beef Top Sirloin, Choice, Lean, Broiled or Braised	3.2
Braised Beef Flank Steak	3.1
Braised Beef Round Steak	3.1
Beef Chuck, Blade Steak, Lean	3.1
Beef Bottom Round, Select, Lean	3.1
Beef Chuck, Stewing Beef, Lean, Trim, Simmered	3.0
Beef Short Loin, T-Bone Steak, Choice, Lean, Broiled	3.0
Beef Bacon, Cooked	2.9
Beef Breakfast Strips, Cured, Cooked	2.9
Beef Chuck, Stewing Beef, Lean and Fat, Simmered	2.8
Beef Top Sirloin, Steak, Lean, Trim, Broiled	2.8

Heme Foods High In Iron

Food Name	Iron (mg/100grams)
Beefalo, Roasted	2.7
Beef Hip, Eye of Round Steak, Lean, Broiled	2.6
Ground Beef, Regular, Baked, Well	2.6
Beef, Cured, Thin Sliced	2.2
Ground Beef, Regular, Pan Fried, Well Done	2.2
Beef Bacon, Lean, Cooked	2.2
Beef Short Loin, Porterhouse Steak, Choice, Broiled	2.2
Beef Pancreas, Braised	2.2
Beef Rib, Whole, Prime, Lean, Roasted	2.2
Lamb	
Lamb Spleen, Raw	41.9
Lamb Spleen, Braised	38.7
Lamb Kidney, Braised	12.4
Lamb Liver, Fried	10.2
Lamb Liver, Braised	8.3
Lamb Liver, Raw	7.4
Lamb Lung, Raw	6.4
Lamb Kidney, Raw	6.4
Lamb Heart, Raw	4.6
Arm Chop, Lean	2 chops =3.4
Lamb Shoulder, Arm, Domestic, Choice, Lean	2.2
Lamb Shoulder, Whole, Domestic, Choice	2.2
Lamb Tongue, Raw or Braised	2.2
Lamb Shoulder, Blade, Domestic, Choice, Lean, Braised	2.2
Braised Lamb Shoulder	2.1
Pork	
Pork Liver, Raw	23.3
Pork Spleen, Raw	22.3
Pork Spleen, Braised	22.2
Pork Lungs, Raw	18.9
Pork Liver, Braised	17.9
Pork Lungs, Braised	16.4

Heme Foods High In Iron

Food Name	Iron (mg/100grams)
Tenderloin, Roasted	6.0
Pork, Loin Chop, Lean and Trimmed	5.8
Sirloin Butt	5.4
Shoulder Butt	2 slices = 5.2
Pork Heart, Raw	4.7
Pork Chitterlings, Simmered	3.7
Pork, Lean Ham, Lean and Trimmed	3.1
Game Meats	
Goat Liver, Fried or Broiled	10.1
Moose Flesh, Dry	9.6
Deer or Venison, Roasted	4.5
Moose, Roasted	4.2
Antelope, Roasted	4.2
Deer or Venison Chops, Cooked	4.1
Goat, Roasted, Backed or Broiled	3.7
Goat Ribs, Cooked	3.7
Goat, Fried	3.5
Elk, Roasted	3.5
Bison (Buffalo), Roasted	3.2
Deer or Venison, Raw	3.2
Moose, Raw	3.1
Antelope, Raw	3.0
Elk, Raw	2.3
Bison, Raw	2.2
Poultry	
Duck Liver, Domesticated, Raw	30.5
Goose Liver, Raw	30.5
Turkey Liver, Raw	10.8
Chicken Liver, Raw	10.6
Chicken Giblets, Fried	10.3
Chicken Heart, Simmered	9.0
Chicken Liver, Simmered	8.5

Heme Foods High In Iron

Food Name	Iron (mg/100grams)
Chicken Liver, Simmered	8.5
Turkey Liver, Simmered	7.8
Chicken, Thigh W/bone	7.5
Turkey Heart, Simmered	6.9
Turkey Giblets, Raw	6.8
Capon Chicken, Giblets, Simmered	6.8
Turkey Giblets, Simmered	6.7
Chicken Giblets, Simmered	6.4
Chicken Heart, Raw	6.0
Chicken Giblets, Raw	5.9
Pintail Duck, Raw	5.3
Turkey Heart, Raw	4.8
Duck Breast, Wild, Meat Only, Raw	4.5
Quail, Meat Only, Raw	4.5
Turkey, dark meat	2.6
Chicken, Breast W/out Bone	2.1
Turkey, white meat	1.6
Chicken, Leg W/bone	1.4
Sea Foods	
Beluga Flesh, Air Dried	91.9
S&W Fine Foods Smoked Baby Clams	35.4
Jonah Crab, Steamed	32.8
Clams, Steamed	31.8
Clams, Mixed Species, Canned, Drained	28.0
Clams, Mixed Species, Cooked, Moist Heat	28.0
Beluga Flesh	25.9
S&W Fine Foods Baby Clams	25.2
Dynasty Whole Baby Clams, Boiled	19.6
Cockles Fish	16.2
Clams, Mixed Species, Raw	14.0
Eulachon (candlefish), Smoked	12.2
Eastern Oyster, Wild, Cooked, Moist Heat	12.0
Cuttlefish, Mixed Species, Cooked, Moist Heat	10.8

Heme Foods High In Iron

Food Name	Iron (mg/100grams)
Whelk, Cooked, Moist Heat	10.1
S&W Fine Foods Oysters	9.6
Octopus, Common, Cooked, Moist Heat	9.5
Pacific Oyster, Cooked, Moist Heat	9.2
Snail or Escargot, Steamed or Poached	9.0
Whitefish, Liver	8.6
Composite-Shellfish, All Types	8.1
Eastern Oyster, Farmed, Cooked, Dry Heat	7.8
Eastern Oyster, Wild, Raw	6.7
Oyster, Baked or Broiled	6.2
Needlefish	6.2
Cuttlefish, Mixed Species, Raw	6.0
Common Octopus, Raw	5.3
Pacific Oyster, Raw	5.1
Whelk, Raw	5.0
Octopus, Raw	4.9
Shrimp, cooked	3.5
Tuna, canned in water	1.7
Flounder, Baked	1.4
Cod, Broiled	1.1
Halibut, cooked	1.1
Salmon, Pink, Canned	1.0

* 100 grams = 1/4 pound or 4 ounces

Appendix B

Non-Heme Foods High In Iron

Food Name	Iron (mg/100grams)
General Mills Total Corn Flakes Cereal	60.0
General Mills Total Whole Grain Cereal	60.0
Kellogg's Product 19 Cereal	60.0
Wheat Flakes Cereal	60.0
Quaker Oats Quick Oats with Iron, Dry	49.5
Wheat Flakes with Raisins Cereal	48.8
Kellogg's Smart Start Cereal	36.0
General Mills Total Raisin Bran Cereal	32.7
Kellogg's Mini Wheats Strawberry Cereal	32.4
Quaker Crunchy Bran Cereal	31.5
Basic Dehydrated Spinach, All Forms	30.6
Kellogg's Mini Wheats Raisin Cereal	30.6
General Mills Total Raisin Bran Cereal	32.7
Kellogg's Mini Wheats Strawberry Cereal	32.4
Quaker Crunchy Bran Cereal	31.5
Basic Dehydrated Spinach, All Forms	30.6
Kellogg's Mini Wheats Raisin Cereal	30.6
General Mills Multi-Bran Chex Cereal	27.9
Popeye Oat'mmms Toasted Oats Cereal	27.9
Post Grape Nuts Flakes Cereal	27.9
Nabisco 100% Bran Cereal	27.9
General Mills Cheerios Cereal	27.0
General Mills Country Corn Flakes Cereal	27.0
General Mills Kaboom Cereal	27.0
General Mills Kix Cereal	27.0
General Mills Wheaties Cereal	27.0
Kellogg's Complete Oat Bran Flakes Cereal	27.0

Non-Heme Foods High In Iron

Food Name	Iron (mg/100grams*)
Kellogg's Just Right Fruit & Nut Cereal	27.0
Kellogg's Special K plus Cereal	27.0
Post Bran Flakes Cereal	27.0
Popeye Oat'mmms Cereal	26.5
Basic Dehydrated Cilantro, All Forms	25.9
Quaker Instant Grits Product with Zesty Cheddar Flavor, Dry	25.7
Quaker Cinnamon Oatmeal Squares Cereal	24.3
Arrowhead Mills Amaranth Flour	24.0
Basic Dehydrated Green Onions, All Forms	22.3
Instant Oatmeal, Fortified, Dry	22.3
Cap'n Crunch Oops! All Berries Cereal	21.8
Dried Agar Seaweed	21.4
Instant Oatmeal with Cinnamon and Spice, Fortified, Dry	21.3
Rice Polish	20.7
Rogers Dehydrated Celery	20.1
Chadler Natural Cocoa Powder	20.0
Basic Freeze Dried Chives, All Forms	19.6
Kettle Sesame Rye with Caraway Organic Tortilla Chips	19.3
Sesame Butter Paste	19.2
Crude Rice Bran	18.5
Total Cereal	1 cup = 18.0
Post Raisin Bran Cereal	18.3
Instant Oatmeal with Bran and Raisins, Fortified, Dry	17.9
Rogers Dehydrated Paprika	17.4
Post Fruity Pebbles Cereal	17.1
Ener-G Gluten Free Potato Flour	16.9
Post Cocoa Pebbles Cereal	16.6
Post Bran Flakes Cereal	16.2
Wheat Bran Cereal	15.9
Quaker Cocoa Blasts Cereal	15.8
Soybeans, Dry or Defatted Flour	1 cup = 15.7
Quaker Marshmallow Safari Cereal	15.0
Dried Pumpkin or Squash Seeds Kernels	15.0
Pumpkin or Squash Seeds, Roasted	14.9

Non-Heme Foods High In Iron

Food Name	Iron (mg/100grams*)
General Mills Crispy Wheaties Raisin Bran Cereal	14.7
Rogers Dehydrated Parsley	14.6
Basic Dehydrated Mushroom, All Forms	14.2
Pumpkin Seeds, Raw	14.4
Tiger's Milk Plus, Powder	1 cup = 14.2
Ralston Wheat Chex	1 cup = 14.0
Life Cereal	1 cup = 12.2
Meat Extender	12.0
Basic Dehydrated Green & White Leeks, All Forms	11.7
Healthy Choice Toasted Brown Sugar Squares Cereal	11.7
Post Fruit & Fibre Dates, Raisins & Walnuts Cereal	11.5
Tofu, Raw, Firm, with Calcium Sulfate	10.5
Ener-G Rice Bran	11.4
Molasses, Black Strap	5 tsp. = 11.3
Rogers Dehydrated Chili Powder with Salt	10.9
Healthy Choice Almond Crunch with Raisins Cereal	10.9
Basic Dehydrated Green Beans, ½" Sliced	10.2
Basic Dehydrated Green Bell Peppers, All Forms	10.1
Post Fruit & Fibre Peaches, Raisins & Almonds Cereal	9.8
Dried Tofu, Frozen	9.7
Dried Tofu, Frozen, Prepared with Calcium	9.7
Lentil Wafers, Broiled	9.6
Beans, Red Kidney, Dry, Uncooked	9.3
Sunflower Seeds	9.3
Raisin Bran Cereal	1 cup = 9.3
US Foods Original Pinto Bean Flakes	9.1
Sunspiced Infused Dried Broccoli, All Forms	8.9
Basic Dehydrated Zucchini, All Forms	8.6
Yardlong Beans	8.6
Basic Dehydrated Celery, All Forms	8.6
Fermented Soy Beans, Mashed	8.6
Basic Dehydrated Mixed Vegetable Blend with Sulfite	8.4

Non-Heme Foods High In Iron

Food Name	Iron (mg/100grams*)
Lemon Grass or Citronella	8.2
Buc Wheat, General Mills	1 cup = 8.0
Quali Tech Flav-r-grain Corn Germ plus Light	8.0
Quali Tech Flav-r-grain Corn Germ, Fine	8.0
Parsley, Raw	8.0
Lima Beans, Dry, Uncooked	7.8
Beans, White, Uncooked	7.8
Beans, Mung, Dry, Uncooked	7.7
Basic Dehydrated Tomatoes, All Forms	7.6
Pink Lentils	7.6
Gebhardt Jalapeno Refried Beans	7.4
Instant Cream of Wheat Cereal, Prepared	7.1
Basic Dehydrated Savoy Cabbage, All Forms	7.1
Potatoes, Skin Only, Baked	7.0
Central Soya Soyarich 115w Soy Flour	7.0
Quali Tech Flav-R-Grain Corn Germ plus	7.0
Chick Peas (Garbanzo) Beans, Dry, Uncooked	6.9
Lentils, Whole, Dry, Uncooked	6.9
Quali Tech Flav-R-Grain P.B.E. Corn Germ	7.0
Spinach, Trimmed Leaves	6.7
Basic Dehydrated Whole Garden Peas	6.6
Basic Dehydrated Beets, Powder	6.9
Beans, Pinto, Calico, Dry Uncooked	6.4
Cornmeal, Whole, Ground	6.3
Beans, Pinto, Gebhardt, Dry Uncooked	6.2
Basic Dehydrated Red Bell Peppers, All Forms	6.0
Adm Sweet N' Neat Raisin Powder	6.0
Basic Fresh Flavor Dehydrated Garlic Products	6.0
California Natural Rice Protein Concentrate 80%	6.0
Rogers Dehydrated Garlic	6.0
Bran, 40%, Fortified	1 cup = 5.6
Instant Cream of Wheat Cereal, Our Original, Prepared	5.5

Non-Heme Foods High In Iron

Food Name	Iron (mg/100grams*)
Tofu, Raw, Regular, with Calcium Sulfate	5.4
Aunt Jemima Buckwheat Pancake Mix	1 cup = 5.4
Peas, Green, Split, Dried, Uncooked	5.1
Peaches, Dry, Uncooked	4.8
Carnation Instant Breakfast	1 serving = 4.6
Wheat Hearts, Cooked with Fat	4.4
Prunes, Dehydrated, Uncooked	8 large
Cream of Wheat Cereal, Cooked	4.3
Spinach, Cooked	1 cup = 4.3
Raisins, Dried, Seedless	4.2
Instant Oatmeal with Raisins and Spice, Fortified, Prepared with Water	4.2
Ovaltine, Low Calorie Mix	1 serving = 4.2
Tofu Rice Burgers (Ovo-lacto)	4.1
Instant Oatmeal with Cinnamon and Spice, Fortified, Prepared with	4.1
Farina Cereal, Cooked with Water	4.1
Wheat and Barley Hot Cereal, Plain or Chocolate, Cooked with Water	4.0
Spinach, Uncooked, Raw	4.0
Instant Oatmeal with Bran and Raisins, Fortified, Prepared with Water	3.9
Coconut Milk	1 cup = 3.9
Composite-instant Hot Cereal	3.8
Cheerios Cereal	1 cup = 3.6
Ener-G Old World Brown Rice Pilaf	3.6
Instant Oatmeal, Fortified, Prepared with Water	3.6
Oat and Grain Hot Cereal, Cooked with Water	3.5
Maple Flavored Oatmeal, Cooked	3.5
Maple and Brown Sugar Instant Oatmeal, Prepared	3.5
Cream of Wheat, Cooked	3.2
Cream of Wheat, Quick or Instant, Prepared with Water and	3.2
Raisins and Spice Instant Oatmeal, Prepared	3.2

Non-Heme Foods High In Iron

Food Name	Iron (mg/100grams*)
Prune Juice	½ cup = 3.0
Watermelon	1 slice = 3.0
Composite-instant or Quick Hot Cereal	3.0
Cream of Wheat, Made with Milk and Sugar, Puerto Rican Style,	2.9
Sugar, Dark Brown	2.9
Potato, Baked, With Skin	1 medium potato = 2.8
Cinnamon and Spice Instant Oatmeal, Prepared	2.7
Cream of Wheat, Cooked with Milk	2.5
Peanut Butter	2.5
Beans, Navy, Cooked	2.3
Peas, Black-Eyed, Cooked	2.2
Multigrain Cereal, Cooked	2.2
Multigrain Cereal, Cooked with Margarine	2.1
Figs, Dried	5 medium = 2.1
Beans, Baked, Canned	2.0
Asparagus, Green, Canned	2.0
Swiss Chard, Cooked	2.0
Rice Krispies Cereal	1 cup = 1.8
Oatmeal, Cooked	1 cup = 1.6
English Muffin	1 whole = 1.6
Spaghetti, Enriched, Cooked	1 cup = 1.6
Bagel	1 whole = 1.5
Peas, Green, Cooked	1 stalk = 1.3
Broccoli, Raw	1.1
Rice, Brown, Cooked	1 cup = 1.0
Whole-Wheat Bread	1 slice = 0.9
Kale, Cooked	0.9
Rice, White, Enriched, Cooked	0.9
Collard Greens, Cooked	0.8
Bread, White	1 slice = 0.7

Non-Heme Foods High In Iron

Food Name	Iron (mg/100grams*)
Broccoli, Cooked	0.6

* 100 grams = 4 ounces or ½ cup approximately.

(This Page Is Purposefully Left Blank For You To Use To Take Notes)

Appendix C

Foods High In Iron

The following list is one that is commonly published. This list indicates foods that are often proposed to be high in iron. At the top of the list are foods which have the highest iron and the lowest calories as we move down the list iron decreases and calories increas2e. This list is now superceded by Appendices A and B what are more accurate. Yet for the most part this list still holds true as a simple and quick reference.

1. Spinach, fresh, cooked
2. Pork, liver, braised
3. Sauerkraut juice, canned
4. Turnip greens, canned
5. Oysters, raw
6. Oysters, smoked
7. Clams, raw
8. Oysters, canned
9. Sauerkraut, canned
10. Clams, canned
11. Lamb, liver, broiled
12. Brewer's Yeast
13. Calf, liver, fried
14. Chicken, liver, simmered
15. Beef, kidneys, cooked
16. Sorghum molasses
17. Clams, meat, steamed
18. Paté, chicken liver, canned
19. beef, heart
20. Turkey, liver, simmered
21. Caviar, sturgeon
22. Beef, liver, braised
23. Pumpkin, canned

24. Oysters, broiled/baked
25. Cherries, sour, red, canned, water
26. Chicken, giblets, simmered
27. Potato, skin, baked
28. Sausage, liver cheese
29. Pork, kidneys, cooked
30. Clams, breaded, fried
31. Oysters, fried
32. Venison, boneless, cooked
33. Bulgur, canned
34. Snails (escargot) w/o shell, cooked
35. Artichoke, cooked
36. Potatoes, instant, mashed
37. Mussels, canned
38. Pumpkin and squash seeds
39. Sardines, canned, mustard sauce
40. Cod, salted, dried
41. Braunschweiger (liver sausage)
42. Wheat germ
43. White beans, cooked
44. Lentils, dry no fat added, cooked

Cereals
1. Total
2. Product 19
3. 40% Bran Flakes, Kellogg's
4. Wheat, puffed, fortified
5. Cream of wheat, cooked

Other Foods High in Iron
1. Beef steak
2. Pine nuts
3. Lima beans, dried
4. Cashew nuts
5. Apricots, peaches, raisins and prunes, dried
6. Kidney beans, dried
7. Turkey, white and dark meats
8. Chicken, white and dark meats

(This Page Is Purposefully Left Blank For You To Use To Take Notes)

Appendix D

Vitamin C and Other Vitamins Supporting Iron Uptake*

Food	Vitamin C (mg)	Vitamin A (IU)	Vitamin D (IU)	Riboflavin (mg)
Basic Dehydrated Red Bell Peppers, All Forms	2051.0	44739.3	0.0	0.8
Basic Dehydrated Green Bell Peppers, All Forms	1852.1	6077.3	0.0	1.2
Basic Dehydrated Mild Green Chili Peppers, All Forms	1852.0	82035.0	0.0	0.7
Basic Freeze Dried Chives, All Forms	978.0	78400.0	0.0	2.2
Basic Dehydrated Parsley, All Forms	735.3	42484.0	0.0	0.9
Basic Dehydrated Lemon Peel, All Forms	659.0	255.0	0.0	0.4
Basic Dehydrated Savoy Cabbage, All Forms	602.1	1604.0	0.0	0.4
Basic Dehydrated Green Onions, All Forms	531.0	59000.0	0.0	1.7
Basic Dehydrated Orange Peel, All Forms	465.0	1436.0	0.0	0.3
Basic Dehydrofrozen Red Bell Peppers, All Cuts	394.8	8612.9	0.0	0.2
Basic Dehydrofrozen Green Chili Peppers, Mild or Hot	378.9	654.8	0.0	0.1
Basic Dehydrated Spinach, All Forms	317.0	75745.0	0.0	2.1
Basic Dehydrated Tomatoes, All Forms	277.9	17890.0	0.0	0.8
Basic Dehydrofrozen Green Bell Peppers, All Cuts	252.1	827.3	0.0	0.2
Basic Dehydrated Mixed Vegetable Blend with Sulfite	240.0	118945.0		0.7
Basic Dehydrated Stew Blend with Sulfite	222.0	28689.0		0.4
Basic Dehydrated Zucchini, All Forms	185.0	6987.0	0.0	0.6
Basic Dehydrated Whole Garden Peas	180.0	2876.0	0.0	0.6
Basic Dehydrated Deluxe Soup Blend with Sulfite	162.0	80066.0		0.6
Basic Dehydrated Green Beans, ½" Sliced	160.1	6560.0	0.0	1.0
Basic Dehydrated Cilantro, All Forms	139.0	36701.0	0.0	1.6
Basic American Potato Pearls Extra Rich	137.0	100.0	0.0	0.2
Basic American Instant Mashed Potatoes, Granules	128.0	100.0	0.0	0.1
Basic American Complete Instant Mashed Potatoes	127.0	100.0	0.0	0.2
Barbados Cherry	126.0	30.0	0.0	0.0
Basic Dehydrated Celery, All Forms	113.0	2276.0	0.0	0.5
Autumn Harvest Orange 100% Juice Base Prepared	91.6	42.6	0.0	
Basic Dehydrated Beets, Powder	83.7	152.0	0.0	0.2
Basic Dehydrated Sweet Potato, All Forms	81.7	72227.0	0.0	0.5
Autumn Harvest Grape 100% Juice Base, Prepared	76.4	5.5	0.0	
Autumn Harvest Apple Juice Base, Prepared	76.0	0.0	0.0	
Autumn Harvest Apple 100% Juice Base, Prepared	75.0	0.0	0.0	

Food	Vitamin C (mg)	Vitamin A (IU)	Vitamin D (IU)	Riboflavin (mg)
Autumn Harvest Cranberry Cocktail Juice Base,	74.3	0.0	0.0	
Autumn Harvest Cranberry Cocktail 50% Juice Base,	74.3	0.0	0.0	
Autumn Harvest Grape Juice Base, Prepared	73.6	5.7	0.0	
Basic Dehydrated Carrots, All Forms	72.4	218858.0	0.0	0.5
Basic Dehydrated Green & White Leeks, All Forms	67.1	531.0	0.0	0.2
Autumn Harvest Cranberry Cocktail 100% Juice Base	66.9	0.0	0.0	
Autumn Harvest Orange Juice Base, Prepared	65.9	135.1	0.0	
Autumn Harvest Prune 100% Juice Base, Prepared	61.1	3.1	0.0	
Autumn Harvest Orange 50% Juice Base, Prepared	57.4	189.9	0.0	
Autumn Harvest Grape 50% Juice Base, Prepared	55.7	4.2	0.0	
Balsam Pear or Bitter Gourd (Peria)	53.0	230.4		0.1
Autumn Harvest Apple 50% Juice Base, Prepared	52.4	0.0	0.0	
Basic American Homestyle Chili Mix Kidney Beans	51.3	100.0		0.3
Bee Pollen	50.0	0.0		0.9
Arizona Mucho Mango Juice Drink	41.7	0.0	0.0	
Basic Dehydrated Mushroom, All Forms	40.0	0.0	0.0	5.1
Barabra's Vanilla Almond Shredded Oats Cereal	38.2	0.0		0.1
Barbara's Shredded Oats Cereal	36.2	0.0		0.1
Adm Supergluten 80 Vital Wheat Gluten	34.5	978.1	30.7	0.3
Apricot Nectar with Added Vitamin C, Canned	33.4	1316.0	0.0	0.0
Banana	31.4	441.7		0.0
Barbara' S Vanilla Animal Cookies	31.0	0.0		
Basic American Potato Slices and Dices, Dry	30.7	100.0	0.0	0.1
Barbara's Cinnamon Puffins Cereal	30.0	0.0		
Basic American Potato Pearls Extra Rich	29.8	112.6	0.0	0.0
Basic Dehydrated Sweet Corn, All Forms	27.4	1132.0	0.0	0.2
Beef and Cheese Quesadilla	27.2	220.1		0.2
Basic American Complete Instant Mashed Potatoes	25.9	56.3		0.0
Asparagus	25.2	140.3		0.1
Banana, Smoked	24.9	39.9		0.4
Arby's Light Menu Garden Salad, No Dressing	24.8			
Basic American Instant Mashed Potatoes Granules	24.5	112.6	0.0	0.0
Asparagus Tips, Frozen, Boiled, Drained	24.4	820.0	0.0	0.1
Basic Fresh Flavor Dehydrated Onion Products	24.0	0.0	0.0	0.7
Barbara's Puffins Cereal	22.2	0.0		
Armour Jumbo Hot Dog	22.0	0.0	36.0	0.1
Beef and Vegetables with Carrots and Broccoli in Soy	21.9	7397.2		0.1
Arby's Light Menu Side Salad, No Dressing	21.6			
Barbara's Bakery Potato Chips, No Salt	21.4	0.0	0.0	
Barbara's Bakery Potato Chips	21.4	0.0	0.0	
Barbara's Bakery Ripple Potato Chips	21.4	0.0	0.0	
Apple Cabbage Slaw	21.0	128.7	2.5	0.0
Arby's Light Menu Roast Chicken Salad	18.7	12.5		0.1
Angela Mia Crushed Tomatoes, Concentrated	18.3	185.7	0.0	
Ambrosia	18.2	290.7	0.0	0.0
Barbara's Organic Soy Essence Cereal	18.0	0.0		

Food	Vitamin C (mg)	Vitamin A (IU)	Vitamin D (IU)	Riboflavin (mg)
Basic American Potato Flakes, Dry	18.0	100.0	0.0	0.1
Barbara's Organic Crispy Wheats Cereal	18.0	0.0		
Basic American Complete Instant Mashed Potatoes	17.6			0.0
Banana, Common Varieties (Pisang)	17.3	501.8		0.1
Barbara's Bakery Cracked Pepper Wheatine	17.1	0.0		
Barbara's Bakery Wheatine Crackers	17.1	0.0		
Barbara's Bakery Yogurt & Green Onion Potato	17.1	0.0	0.0	
Barbara's Bakery Sesame Wheatine Crackers	17.1	0.0		
Beef Flauta or Taquito	17.0	187.1		0.1
Basic American Potato Pearls Extra Rich, Dry	16.6	100.0	0.0	0.2
Arby's Broccoli 'N Cheddar Baked Potato	16.6	13.0		0.1
Balsamic Tomato Salad	16.1	524.0	0.0	0.1
Barbara's Old Fashioned Oatmeal Crisp Cookies	15.0	0.0		
Barbara's Shredded Spoonfuls Cereal	15.0	0.0		
Baked Crispy Potatoes	14.6	13.7	0.0	0.0
Banana (Pisang Nangka)	14.1	330.7		0.1
Baked Rosemary Chicken with Broccoli & Carrots	14.0	5647.8	0.0	0.1
Bean Dip, Made with Refried Beans	13.6	289.2		0.1
Baked Sweet Potatoes and Apples	13.5	4123.9	8.0	0.0
Arby' S Homestyle Fries	13.3			
Angela Mia Pear Shaped Tomatoes	12.7	67.4	0.0	
Artichoke, Edible Parts	12.5	0.0	0.0	0.1
Arizona Crazy Cocktail Juice Drink	12.5	1041.7		
Banana (Pisang Abu)	12.1	70.0		0.0
Beef and Vegetable Fajita	12.0	192.7		0.1
Angela Mia Chopped Tomatoes	11.8	150.4	0.0	
Banquet Chicken Parmigiana Meal	11.1	37.1		
Acorn Squash	11.0	339.5		0.0
Asparagus Tips, Boiled, Drained	10.8	540.0	0.0	0.1
Acorn Squash, Baked	10.8	428.1		0.0
Barbecue Sauce	10.7	704.7	0.0	0.1
Asparagus, Canned	10.6	0.0		0.1
Baked Beans with Franks	10.5	240.7	3.5	0.0
Arizona Total Sport Extreme Thirst Quencher Lemon	10.4	520.8	0.0	
Arby's Baked Potato with Butter & Sour Cream	10.3			
Baked Potato/Marinara with Tofu (Vegan)	10.1	275.1	0.0	0.0
Au Gratin Potatoes	10.1	289.6		0.1
Applesauce, Unsweetened, Canned	10.0	29.0	0.0	0.0
Avocado Pear	10.0	330.7		0.4
Arby's Deluxe Baked Potato	9.5	14.3		0.0
Bean Deep Fried Burrito, Cheese, Lettuce, Tomato	9.4	489.9		0.1
Angela Mia Crushed Tomatoes	9.3	130.6	0.0	
Banana Foster	9.2	59.6	0.0	0.1
Beef and Bean Deep Fried Burrito with Lettuce and	9.1	339.8		0.1
Banana	9.1	81.3	0.0	0.1
Asparagus, Trimmed Ends	9.1	614.6	0.0	0.1

Food	Vitamin C (mg)	Vitamin A (IU)	Vitamin D (IU)	Riboflavin (mg)
Bacon, Lettuce and Tomato Sandwich Mayonnaise	8.9	315.7		0.2
Banana	8.7	55.5	0.0	0.1
Aloe Vera Vegetable Juice	8.5	50.0	0.0	0.1
Arby's Curly Fries	8.5	50.5	0.0	0.1
Basic American Potato Slices and Dices, Rehydrated	8.5	138.9	0.0	0.0
Beef and Rice Soup, Puerto Rican Style	8.4	125.3		0.1
Banana (Pisang Mas)	8.3	632.5		0.1
Avocado, California	8.2	75.1	0.0	0.2
Baked Salmon with Cucumber Dill Sauce	8.0	119.0	0.0	0.1
Avocado, Non California	7.9	612.0	0.0	0.1
Asparagus Pasta Stir Fry (Vegan)	7.9	384.3	0.0	0.1
Baked Celery, Almonds and Broccoli (Lacto)	7.8	795.9	4.4	0.1
Avocado Dip (Guacamole)	7.7	459.9	9.5	0.1
Ball Park Fat Free Frank	7.2	0.0		
Ball Park Fat Free Smoke White Turkey Frank	7.2	0.0	11.8	
Ball Park Lite Frank	7.2	0.0		
Basic American Golden Grill Hashbrowns	7.1	192.3	0.0	0.0
Arby's Cream of Broccoli Soup	7.1	352.1		0.2
Arby's Cheddar Curly Fries	7.1	35.4		0.1
Bamboo Shoots (Rebung)	7.0	30.0		0.0
Nonfat Dry Milk	6.8	26.7		1.6
Basic American Redi-shred Hashbrowns	6.7	192.3	0.0	0.1
Bean Taco or Tostada with Lettuce, Tomato, Salsa	6.7	267.0		0.1
Acorn Squash, Boiled, Mashed	6.5	257.1		0.0
Ball Park Beef Frank	6.4	0.0		
Beef Burritos	6.3	218.2	0.0	0.1
Beef and Bean Tamale Pie	6.3	529.4	5.1	0.2
Bean Taco or Tostada, Cheese, Lettuce, Tomato	6.2	321.3		0.1
Baked Onions	6.1	98.6	0.0	0.0
Beef and Potatoes (Carne con Papas)	5.8	145.2	0.0	0.2
Banana (Pisang Kari)	5.8	371.0		0.0
Apple with Skin	5.7	52.9	0.0	0.0
Baked Chili Relleno (Ovo-Lacto)	5.5	570.6	12.1	0.2
Beef Burrito	5.1	702.1	3.0	0.2
Beef Deep Fried Burrito, Cheese, Lettuce, Tomato	5.0	345.1		0.2
Baked Apple with Liquid, Unsweetened	4.9	48.4	0.0	0.0
Bean Taco	4.9	381.1	1.1	0.1
Barbecued Chicken	4.5	263.5	0.0	0.1
Baked Stuffed Cod	4.2	246.6	56.4	0.1
Apricot Pie, 2 Crusts	4.1	1137.5		0.1
Banana Fritter	4.0	227.2		0.2
Barbara's Bakery Brown Rice Crisps Cereal	4.0	0.0		
Arby's Lumberjack Mixed Vegetable Soup	3.9	1100.4		0.0
Baked Beans	3.9	227.7	0.0	0.1
Antipasto with Ham, Fish, Cheese and Vegetables	3.9	4765.7		0.2
Barracuda Fillet, Baked or Broiled	3.7	172.9		0.5

Food	Vitamin C (mg)	Vitamin A (IU)	Vitamin D (IU)	Riboflavin (mg)
Baked Fish Fillets	3.6	36.5	63.8	0.1
Baked Spicy Fish	3.3	358.2	56.7	0.1
Baked Flounder	3.2	183.0	13.2	0.1
Arby's Italian Sub Sandwich	3.1	17.2		0.2
Beans with Vegetable Rice	3.0	5263.9	0.0	0.1
Beef and Potato Gordita with Lettuce and Salsa	3.0	143.1	0.0	0.1
Baked Beans, Canned	3.0	1501.8		0.1
Beef and Bean Nachos with Cheese and Sour Cream	3.0	348.4		0.2
Abalone, Steamed or Poached	3.0	8.9		0.1
Arby's Turkey Sub Sandwich	3.0	16.5		0.1
Arby's Roast Beef Sub Sandwich	2.9	16.5		0.2
Arizona Kiwi Strawberry Juice Drink	2.9	0.0	0.0	
Basic American Potato Flakes, Rehydrated	2.9	90.9	0.0	0.1
Bearitos Fat Free Original Baked Beans	2.8	153.8	0.0	
Atlantic Snow, Spider or Queen Crab, Canned, Drained	2.7	6.7		0.1
Banana Loaf	2.6	82.2	6.3	0.2
Angostura Soy Sauce	2.6	0.0	0.0	
Arby's Arby-Q Sandwich	2.6	26.9		
Angostura Teriyaki Sauce	2.4	0.0	0.0	
Apricot Flavored Yogurt	2.4	295.1		0.3
Banana Nut Bread	2.4	262.2	2.6	0.4
Arroz Con Queso (Rice With Cheese) (Lacto)	2.3	207.4	4.2	0.1
Beans	2.3	63.7	0.0	0.1
Angela Mia Crushed Tomatoes	2.3	166.1	0.0	
Bamboo Shoots, Braised, Canned	2.2	180.2		0.0
Apple Juice, Frozen Concentrate	2.1	0.0	0.0	0.1
Baked Beans with Pork, Canned	2.0	177.6		0.0
Apples in Heavy Syrup, Canned	2.0	50.0		0.0

* 100 grams = 4 ounces or ½ cup approximately.

(This Page Is Purposefully Left Blank For You To Use To Take Notes)

Appendix E

Vitamin A and Other Vitamins Supporting Iron Uptake*

Food	Vitamin A (IU)	Vitamin C (mg)	Vitamin D (IU)	Riboflavin (mg)
Basic Dehydrated Carrots, All Forms	218858.0	72.4	0.0	0.5
Basic Dehydrated Mixed Vegetable Blend with Sulfite	118945.0	240.0		0.7
Basic Dehydrated Mild Green Chili Peppers, All Forms	82035.0	1852.0	0.0	0.7
Basic Dehydrated Deluxe Soup Blend with Sulfite	80066.0	162.0		0.6
Basic Freeze Dried Chives, All Forms	78400.0	978.0	0.0	2.2
Basic Dehydrated Spinach, All Forms	75745.0	317.0	0.0	2.1
Basic Dehydrated Sweet Potato, All Forms	72227.0	81.7	0.0	0.5
Basic Dehydrated Green Onions, All Forms	59000.0	531.0	0.0	1.7
Basic Dehydrated Red Bell Peppers, All Forms	44739.3	2051.0	0.0	0.8
Basic Dehydrated Parsley, All Forms	42484.0	735.3	0.0	0.9
Basic Dehydrated Cilantro, All Forms	36701.0	139.0	0.0	1.6
Basic Dehydrated Stew Blend with Sulfite	28689.0	222.0		0.4
Basic Dehydrated Tomatoes, All Forms	17890.0	277.9	0.0	0.8
Basic Dehydrofrozen Red Bell Peppers, All Cuts	8612.9	394.8	0.0	0.2
Beef and Vegetables with Carrots and Broccoli in Soy	7397.2	21.9		0.1
Basic Dehydrated Zucchini, All Forms	6987.0	185.0	0.0	0.6
Basic Dehydrated Green Beans, ½" Sliced	6560.0	160.1	0.0	1.0
Basic Dehydrated Green Bell Peppers, All Forms	6077.3	1852.1	0.0	1.2
Baked Rosemary Chicken with Broccoli & Carrots	5647.8	14.0	0.0	0.1
Beans with Vegetable & Rice	5263.9	3.0	0.0	0.1
Baked Sweet Potatoes and Apples	4123.9	13.5	8.0	0.0
Basic Dehydrated Whole Garden Peas	2876.0	180.0	0.0	0.6
Beef Curry (Kari Daging Lembu)	2420.5	0.0		0.1
Basic Dehydrated Celery, All Forms	2276.0	113.0	0.0	0.5
Beef Burger (Burger Daging Lembu)	1943.5	0.0		0.1
Beach Glasswort Asparagus	1927.3	1.8	0.0	0.1
Beef Burger Patty (Burger Daging Lembu)	1919.7	0.9		0.2
Basic Dehydrated Savoy Cabbage, All Forms	1604.0	602.1	0.0	0.4
Banquet Roasted White Turkey Meal	1567.7	1.4		
Baked Beans, Canned	1501.8	3.0		0.1
Basic Dehydrated Orange Peel, All Forms	1436.0	465.0	0.0	0.3
Apricot Nectar with Added Vitamin C, Canned	1316.0	33.4	0.0	0.0
Bandung Style Rice Noodles (Mee-hoon Bandung)	1247.4	0.0		0.1
Bandung Style Rice Noodles (Kuih-teow Bandung)	1236.7	0.0		0.1
Bandung Style Wheat Noodles (Mee Bandung)	1236.7	0.0		0.1
Bearitos Low Fat Black Bean Premium Chili	1224.5	3.7		

Vitamin A and Other Vitamins Supporting Iron Uptake*

Food	Vitamin A (IU)	Vitamin C (mg)	Vitamin D (IU)	Riboflavin (mg)
Basic Dehydrated Sweet Corn, All Forms	1132.0	27.4	0.0	0.2
Arby's Lumberjack Mixed Vegetable Soup	1100.4	3.9		0.0
Arctic Char, Raw	1099.9	0.0		0.3
Arizona Crazy Cocktail Juice Drink	1041.7	12.5		
Banquet Homestyle Noodles and Chicken Meal	1028.8	0.0		
Banquet Chicken Pasta Primavera Meal	928.2	0.0		
Banana	830.4	16.3		0.1
Basic DehydroFrozen Green Bell Peppers, All Cuts	827.3	252.1	0.0	0.2
Asparagus Tips, Frozen, Boiled, Drained	820.0	24.4	0.0	0.1
Bearitos Mexican Style Beans & Rice	816.3	2.4		
Baked Celery, Almonds and Broccoli (Lacto)	795.9	7.8	4.4	0.1
Bearitos Cuban Style Beans & Rice	714.3	6.1		
Bearitos White or Yellow Tortilla Chips, No Salt	714.3	0.0	0.0	
Barbecue Sauce	704.7	10.7	0.0	0.1
Beef Burrito	702.1	5.1	3.0	0.2
Bacon, Egg and Cheese Croissant Sandwich	698.5	1.4	32.0	0.4
Apricot Buttermilk	695.2	0.8	0.0	0.1
Bean Burrito	683.5	5.5	2.9	0.2
Basic DehydroFrozen Green Chili Peppers, Mild or	654.8	378.9	0.0	0.1
Asparagus, Trimmed Ends	614.6	9.1	0.0	0.1
Bearitos Cajun Style Beans & Rice	612.2	2.4		
Avocado	612.0	7.9	0.0	0.1
Baked Chili Relleno (Ovo-Lacto)	570.6	5.5	12.1	0.2
Asparagus Tips, Boiled, Drained	540.0	10.8	0.0	0.1
Basic Dehydrated Green & White Leeks, All Forms	531.0	67.1	0.0	0.2
Balsamic Tomato Salad	524.0	16.1	0.0	0.1
ARIZONA Total Sport Extreme Thirst Quencher	520.8	10.4	0.0	
Bearitos Low Fat Spicy Premium Chili	510.2	6.1		
Bearitos Low Fat Original Premium Chili	510.2	6.1		
Banana, Common Varieties (Pisang)	501.8	17.3		0.1
Bean Deep Fried Burrito with Cheese, Lettuce and	489.9	9.4		0.1
Avocado Dip (Guacamole)	459.9	7.7	9.5	0.1
Arby's Old Fashioned Chicken Noodle Soup	440.1	0.3		0.0
Acorn Squash, Baked	428.1	10.8		0.0
Banquet Fried Rice with Chicken & Egg Rolls Meal	415.0	0.0		
Asparagus Pasta Stir Fry (Vegan)	384.3	7.9	0.0	0.1
Bean Taco	381.1	4.9	1.1	0.1
Bean Soup	350.1	1.2	0.0	0.1
Acorn Squash	339.5	11.0		0.0
Avocado Pear	330.7	10.0		0.4
Baked Beans	312.2	1.7	0.0	0.1
Aunt Jemima Yellow Corn Meal Mix, Self Rising	289.7	0.0	0.0	0.6
Au Gratin Potatoes	289.6	10.1		0.1
Bean Dip, Made with Refried Beans	289.2	13.6		0.1
Baked Macaroni and Cheese	285.8	0.4	22.6	0.2

Vitamin A and Other Vitamins Supporting Iron Uptake*				
Food	Vitamin A (IU)	Vitamin C (mg)	Vitamin D (IU)	Riboflavin (mg)
100% Whole Grain Waffle	266.0	0.6		0.3
Armour Lowfat Milk Replacer	265.6	1.6		1.7
Barbecued Chicken	263.5	4.5	0.0	0.1
Acorn Squash, Boiled, Mashed	257.1	6.5		0.0
BASIC Dehydrated Lemon Peel, All Forms	255.0	659.0	0.0	0.4
AUNT JEMIMA White Corn Meal, Self Rising,	205.0	0.0	0.0	0.4
Baked Flounder	183.0	3.2	13.2	0.1
Barracuda Fillet, Baked or Broiled	172.9	3.7		0.5
Atlantic and Pacific Halibut, Raw	155.0	0.0	188.0	0.1
Beef Burger	145.2	0.6		0.1
Asparagus	140.3	25.2		0.1
Autumn Harvest Orange Juice Base, Prepared	135.1	65.9	0.0	
Angela Mia Crushed Tomatoes	130.6	9.3	0.0	
Angela Mia Marinara Sauce	129.6	6.2	0.0	
Avocado, California	75.1	8.2	0.0	0.2
Aloe Vera Vegetable Juice	50.0	8.5	0.0	0.1
Baked Apple with Liquid, Unsweetened	48.4	4.9	0.0	0.0
Barracuda, Steamed or Poached	46.3	1.9		0.5
Atlantic Cod or Scrod, Baked or Broiled	45.8	1.0		0.1
Apple without Skin, Sliced, Boiled	44.1	0.2	0.0	0.0
Atlantic Cod or Scrod, Raw	40.0	1.0	44.0	0.1
Applesauce	19.2	1.8	0.0	0.0
Applesauce, Sweetened, Canned	11.0	1.7	0.0	0.0
Applesauce, Sweetened with Sugar	11.0	1.7	0.0	0.0
Apples, Pureed (Manzana Puré)	10.0	1.0	0.0	0.0

* 100 grams = 4 ounces or ½ cup approximately.

(This Page Is Purposefully Left Blank For You To Use To Take Notes)

Appendix F

Vitamin D and Other Vitamins Supporting Iron Uptake*

Food	Vitamin D (IU)	Vitamin C (mg)	Vitamin A (IU)	Riboflavin (mg)
Atlantic Smelt, Canned	300.0	0.0	96.0	
Atlantic Sardine with Bone, Canned in Oil, Drained	272.0	0.0	224.0	0.2
Atlantic and Pacific Halibut, Raw	188.0	0.0	155.0	0.1
Baked Fish Fillets	63.8	3.6	36.5	0.1
Baked Cod with Cheese	59.5	1.1	135.5	0.1
Baked Spicy Fish	56.7	3.3	358.2	0.1
Baked Stuffed Cod	56.4	4.2	246.6	0.1
Atlantic Cod or Scrod, Raw	44.0	1.0	40.0	0.1
Baked Custard	41.1	0.8	279.8	0.2
Armour Jumbo Hot Dog	36.0	22.0	0.0	0.1
Baked French Toast	32.7	0.4	242.1	0.3
Bacon and Egg Croissant Sandwich	32.0	1.3	607.3	0.3
Bacon, Egg and Cheese Croissant Sandwich	32.0	1.4	698.5	0.4
Apple Honey Crisp	28.6	0.7	337.2	0.1
Apple Crisp	28.6	0.7	337.2	0.1
Baked Macaroni and Cheese	22.6	0.4	285.8	0.2
Baking Powder Biscuits	13.6	0.2	73.3	0.3
Baked Flounder	13.2	3.2	183.0	0.1
Barley Pilaf	12.5	1.6	50.3	0.1
Applesauce Cake	12.2	0.9	120.6	0.2
Baked Chili Relleno (Ovo-Lacto)	12.1	5.5	570.6	0.2
Banana Bread Squares (Master Mix)	11.8	2.5	125.1	0.2
Ball Park Fat Free Smoke White Turkey Frank	11.8	7.2	0.0	
Baking Powder Biscuits (Master Mix)	11.0	0.1	59.1	0.2
Apple Cobbler	10.9	0.3	135.3	0.0
Baked Macaroni and Cheese with Eggs (Ovo-Lacto)	9.8	0.2	252.3	0.1
Avocado Dip (Guacamole)	9.5	7.7	459.9	0.1
Baked Meatballs	9.4	0.4	73.6	0.3
Baked Sweet Potatoes and Apples	8.0	13.5	4123.9	0.0
Baker's Real Milk Chocolate Chips	7.7	0.0	0.0	0.2
Banana Cream Tart	7.4	4.3	74.9	0.1
Banana Loaf	6.3	2.6	82.2	0.2
Banana Bread Squares	6.2	2.5	96.8	0.2
Beef and Bean Tamale Pie	5.1	6.3	529.4	0.2
Atole	5.1	0.2	14.4	0.0
Aunt Jemima Buttermilk Complete Pancake & Waffle Mix	5.0	0.1	48.2	0.4

Vitamin D and Other Vitamins Supporting Iron Uptake*				
Food	Vitamin D (IU)	Vitamin C (mg)	Vitamin A (IU)	Riboflavin (mg)
Baked Celery, Almonds and Broccoli (Lacto)	4.4	7.8	795.9	0.1
Arroz Con Queso (Rice With Cheese) (Lacto)	4.2	2.3	207.4	0.1
Aunt Jemima Reduced Calorie Buttermilk Complete	4.2	0.3	68.0	1.0
Baked Beans with Franks	3.5	10.5	240.7	0.0
Beef Burrito	3.0	5.1	702.1	0.3
Bean Burrito	2.9	5.5	683.5	0.2
Apple-Spice Snack Cake	2.6	0.5	42.5	0.2
Banana Nut Bread	2.6	2.4	262.2	0.4
Apple Cabbage Slaw	2.5	21.0	128.7	0.0

* 100 grams = 4 ounces or ½ cup approximately.

Appendix G

Riboflavin (Vitamin B2) and Other Vitamins Supporting Iron Uptake*

Food	Riboflavin (mg)	Vitamin C (mg)	Vitamin A (IU)	Vitamin D (IU)
Beef Extract	6.9	0.0	160.2	
Baker's Yeast, Active, Dry	5.4	0.3	1.0	0.0
Basic Dehydrated Mushroom, All Forms	5.1	40.0	0.0	0.0
Basic Freeze Dried Chives, All Forms	2.2	978.0	78400.0	0.0
Basic Dehydrated Spinach, All Forms	2.1	317.0	75745.0	0.0
Armour Lowfat Milk Replacer	1.7	1.6	265.6	
Adm Aytex P Wheat Starch	1.7	0.6	0.0	0.0
Basic Dehydrated Green Onions, All Forms	1.7	531.0	59000.0	0.0
Basic Dehydrated Cilantro, All Forms	1.6	139.0	36701.0	0.0
Baker's Yeast, Compressed	1.3	0.1	0.0	0.0
Basic Dehydrated Green Bell Peppers, All Forms	1.2	1852.1	6077.3	0.0
Basic Dehydrated Green Beans, ½" Sliced	1.0	160.1	6560.0	0.0
Aunt Jemima Reduced Calorie Buttermilk Complete	1.0	0.3	68.0	4.2
Aunt Jemima Whole Wheat Pancake & Waffle Mix	0.9	0.0	16.3	0.0
Basic Dehydrated Parsley, All Forms	0.9	735.3	42484.0	0.0
Bee Pollen	0.9	50.0	0.0	
Aunt Jemima Buttermilk White Corn Meal Mix, Self	0.8	0.0	2.2	0.0
Basic Dehydrated Red Bell Peppers, All Forms	0.8	2051.0	44739.3	0.0
Basic Dehydrated Tomatoes, All Forms	0.8	277.9	17890.0	0.0
Basic Fresh Flavor Dehydrated Onion Products	0.7	24.0	0.0	0.0
Basic Dehydrated Mild Green Chili Peppers, All	0.7	1852.0	82035.0	0.0
Bean Flour (Harina de Frijol)	0.7	0.0	0.0	0.0
Basic Dehydrated Mixed Vegetable Blend with Sulfite	0.7	240.0	118945.	
Aunt Jemima Yellow Corn Meal Mix, Self Rising	0.6	0.0	289.7	0.0
Basic Dehydrated Deluxe Soup Blend with Sulfite	0.6	162.0	80066.0	
Basic Dehydrated Zucchini, All Forms	0.6	185.0	6987.0	0.0
Basic Dehydrated Whole Garden Peas	0.6	180.0	2876.0	0.0
Basic Dehydrated Celery, All Forms	0.5	113.0	2276.0	0.0
Basic Dehydrated Sweet Potato, All Forms	0.5	81.7	72227.0	0.0
Almonds	0.5	1.7	0.0	

* 100 grams = 4 ounces or ½ cup approximately.

(This Page Is Purposefully Left Blank For You To Use To Take Notes)

Prescription And Over-The-Counter Iron Products

Iron Preparations Are Sold Under The Following Names*:

Slo-Fe, Feosol, Fero-Grad, Ferrous Sulfate, Ferrous Fumerate, Ferrous Gluconate, Nephro-Fer, Hemocyte, Chem-Sol, Fe-Mar, Fe-Max, Fer-Gen-Sol, Fersul, Ferra-Tab, Ferra-TD, Ferro-Time, Ironmar, Iron Sol, Plexafer, Siderol plus many products combines with Folic acid and other combinations of vitamins and minerals.

Each of the above products are either ferrous sulfate, gluconate or fumerate and are used for the treatment of iron deficiency and Iron Deficiency Anemia. Used as directed over time they can produce a significant reduction in the incidence of the most common side effects associated with iron deficiency anemia.

Each tablet contains between 160 mg and 325 mg of ferrous iron.

Warnings

The treatment of any iron preparation should always be under the care, advice and supervision of a legally licenced physician. Since iron products interfere with absorption of oral tetracycline antibiotics, these products should not be taken within 2 hours of each other. As with any drug, if you are pregnant or nursing a baby, seek the advice of a health professional before using this product. Accidental overdose of iron-containing products is a leading cause of fatal poisoning in children under 6 years of age, there fore it is important to KEEP THESE PRODUCTS OUT OF REACH OF CHILDREN. In case of accidental overdose, call a doctor or poison control center immediately.

Dosage And Administration

Adults One (1) or 2 tablets daily or as recommended by a physician. A maximum of 4 tablets daily may be taken. Children One (1) tablet daily or as prescribed by the physician. Tablets must be swallowed whole.

* Most common brand names used for iron sold in the U.S.A.

One Week Sample Menu

	Sunday	Monday	Tuesday	Wednesday	Thursday	Friday	Saturday
Breakfast							
AM Snack							
Lunch							
Afternoon Snack							
Dinner							
PM Snack							

End Notes

1. *Hemoglobin* is actually an oxygen carrying red pigment which makes up red blood cells. It is made up of two major components a protein molecule called *globin* and the iron component called *heme*, hence *hemoglobin*. In its ordinary form, when it combines with oxygen it is often called *oxyhemoglobin*.

2. *Ferritin* is an iron-protein compound which is found in many different tissues of the body, it holds and stores iron a large portion of the iron stored in the body.

3. *Hemosiderin* is a dark yellow pigment which is made from the iron portion of degenerating red blood cells. It is the second most common way that iron is stored in the body waiting to be reused to make new hemoglobin. It is most commonly found in immune system cells called phagocytes circulating in the blood stream.

4. *Macrophages* are large cells that wander freely through the body looking for, finding and destroying foreign bodies, and invaders such as bacteria and viruses.

5. *Mean Corpuscular Volume* (MCV) is the average volume of a single red cell as measured by an automated test which works by electrical impedance, or by light scatter. It is generally increased in liver disease, folate and B12 deficiency anemias and during use of certain drugs methotrexate, phenytoin, zidovudine. It is usually decreased in IDA, thalassemia and during anemia of chronic disease.

6. *Mean Corpuscular Hemoglobin* (MCH) is the amount of hemoglobin in each red blood cell in absolute units. A low MCH can mean hypochromic anemia or microcytosis or both. A high MCH is evidence of enlarged red blood cells (macrocytosis). Decreased MCH is found in IDA and thalassemia). The MCH is calculated from the measured values of hemoglobin (Hb) and red cell count (RBC) by a specific formula.

7. *Mean Corpuscular Hemoglobin Concentration* (MCHC) describes how filled the red cell volume is filled with hemoglobin. It is calculated from the measured hemoglobin (Hb), the mean corpuscular volume (MCV), and red cell count (RBC) by a specific formula. MCHC is decreased in IDA , thalassemia, lead poisoning), and the anemia caused by chronic diseases.

8. *Hypochromic* (or hypochromia) refers to the fact that the cells are no longer bright red, but rather lighter in color or even a light pink. They are deficient in hemoglobin the red pigment that carries oxygen. The term microcytic refers to the fact that these anemic red blood cells are nor reduced in size, smaller than normal, hence micro (small) and cytic (cells).

9. By low *transferrin saturation* (TIBC), we refer to the fact that transferrin is a protein molecule found in the blood, it transports iron and controls the amounts

and location of iron is in the body. When the transferrin saturation is low it is an indication of IDA.

10.   *Thalassemia* is a hereditary type of anemia which is found primarily in individuals with roots in the Mediterranean and surrounding area and South East Asia. There are two sub groups Thalassemia major and Thalassemia minor. It can be lethal and must be differentiated from the milder IDA.

11.   *Cognitive capacity* refers to an individual's awareness, perception of what is happening around him or her, reasoning ability, judgement, intuition, and memory. Ones ability to understand and correctly interpret the world around them is based on their cognitive capacity. A person who has normal cognitive development has normally functioning mental processes, can reasonably correctly interpret events around them and has insight and understanding of them self and the world around them.

12.   The *extrusion reflex* is and infantile reflex during which the tongue moves outward or out of the mouth after it has been touched. It is generally present in healthy babies from birth to the end of the fourth month.

13.   Unfortunately once any diagnostic laboratory test is read as "*outside of the normal range,*" additional diagnostic testing is usually needed to either confirm or deny a diagnosis of anemia and determine the exact type of anemia. If all, or most, of these tests are outside of the normal range, and the finding are consistent with medical history and even physical examination, then the original testing can then be considered clearly to be abnormal. On the other hand, if the most important of these tests are "normal," then those that are still abnormal (after all other reasons why they might be abnormal have been ruled out) will tell us that this person is in fact normal even with sightly abnormal values in some of the test. In the end, the final determination will have to be based on whether the person is healthy and fully functional in all other ways.